Strong Roots

Strong Roots:

Terrain-Based ALS Support for Patients and Families

By Riley McPherson

ISBN: 979-8-9990723-1-3

Printed in the United States

This book is for educational and informational purposes only. It is not intended to diagnose, treat, cure, or prevent any disease, nor should it be used as a substitute for medical advice from a qualified healthcare professional. The author is not a licensed medical doctor, and the content herein is based on independent research, published scientific literature, clinical experience, and terrain-based frameworks for healing.

Readers are encouraged to consult with their healthcare providers before making any changes to diet, supplements, medications, or treatment plans, especially in the context of complex conditions such as ALS or other neurodegenerative diseases.

The author and publisher disclaim any liability arising directly or indirectly from the use or misuse of the information presented in this book. The reader assumes full responsibility for any outcomes resulting from actions taken based on this content.

"What lies behind us and what lies before us are tiny matters compared to what lies within us."

Ralph Waldo Emerson

Table of Content

Introduction

An ALS diagnosis often lands like an avalanche. There's shock, fear, and the heavy thud of urgency that follows. Appointments are scheduled quickly, explanations are clinical, and the words that surface most often are the ones no one wants to hear: progressive, irreversible, terminal. It's easy, in that moment, to feel like the ground has disappeared.

But this book is not written from that place of panic. It's written from a quieter space, one where there is time to breathe, observe, and begin again. A space that recognizes that the body is not broken beyond hope. It is dysregulated, depleted, and overwhelmed, but still responding, still adapting, still communicating.

Rather than focusing on deterioration, this book focuses on possibility. Not false hope. Not magical thinking. But real, steady support for the internal terrain that has been breaking down long before a diagnosis was named.

ALS is not just a disease of the motor neurons. It is a collapse of multiple systems: digestion, drainage, mitochondrial energy, immune regulation, and nervous system safety. And when we look at it through this lens, through the interconnected patterns of breakdown, we can also begin to trace the shape of healing.

This doesn't mean a quick fix. It doesn't promise reversal. But it offers something essential that many people lose in the clinical fog: the ability to participate in your care with intelligence, agency, and compassion. To support the body in ways that do not overwhelm it further. To shift the question from "What's the prognosis?" to "What does my terrain need now?"

This book exists because the current conversation around ALS is too narrow. It leaves people without tools, without time, and too often, without dignity. Here, we begin a new conversation, one rooted in clarity, curiosity, and care.

The Problem with Standard Approaches

Conventional medicine approaches ALS as a disease of the nervous system, specifically, as a progressive and untreatable breakdown of motor neurons. The focus is almost entirely on what's being lost: muscle function, mobility, speech, independence. Most treatments offered are aimed at slowing this decline or managing its symptoms, breathing machines, feeding tubes, pharmaceutical interventions to blunt progression by a few months. This model, while technologically advanced, is still profoundly narrow.

It tends to see the body in pieces. It treats muscles as separate from mitochondria, the nervous system as separate from digestion, and immune activity as a threat rather than a response. The result is a system of care that becomes about managing decline rather than understanding the conditions that caused that decline in the first place.

What's missing in this model isn't just a cure. What's missing is a whole paradigm: one that sees the body as an interconnected terrain.

In this terrain view, ALS doesn't begin with a twitch or stumble. It begins much earlier, when the gut lining starts to leak, when mitochondria lose their capacity to produce clean energy, when toxins build up faster than they can be cleared, when chronic infections go silent but not inactive, when trauma lodges itself in the tissues and begins to alter physiology.

Mainstream care rarely addresses these root issues. It doesn't ask why the terrain broke down, only how to slow what's already in motion. And for many patients, this creates a kind of emotional exile. You're given a name, but not a path. You're handed expectations, but not meaningful tools.

This book is different. It honors what's missing from the standard model: nourishment, rhythm, coherence, and respect for the body's deep intelligence. Because ALS is not just a disease of the nervous system. It is a systemic collapse of boundaries, signals, and repair. And when we support the terrain, we support everything, because everything is connected.

A Terrain-Based Philosophy of Healing

When we talk about "terrain," we're talking about the body's internal ecosystem, the soil in which all health or disease grows. It's not one organ or one function. It's the sum of everything: your gut lining, your mitochondria, your immune signaling, your circulation, your fascia and lymph, your emotional resilience, your nervous system tone. It's the invisible web of relationships that determines how well your body can adapt, repair, and defend itself.

In ALS, this terrain is not simply damaged, it's overwhelmed. The gut may be inflamed and leaky, allowing immune-disruptive fragments into circulation. Mitochondria may be underpowered, unable to generate clean energy. Toxins, environmental, microbial, emotional, may be building up faster than the body can process or release them. And the nervous system may be trapped in a state of chronic alert, unable to downshift into healing.

It's a perfect storm. And yet, each part of that storm is responsive. Each system can be supported, if we listen carefully and proceed with respect.

This philosophy doesn't begin with killing pathogens or pulling metals from the body. It doesn't start with force. It starts with nourishment. With restoring rhythm. With stabilizing what's already struggling. A dehydrated, underfed, sleep-deprived, emotionally frayed body cannot detox. It cannot regenerate. It can only protect itself, and in ALS, that protective mode often looks like collapse.

So we begin at the root. We calm what's overactive. We feed what's depleted. We open what's stagnant. We don't try to override the body, we try to support its return to coherence. This is the terrain model: slow, layered, intelligent, and deeply personal.

Healing doesn't begin with fighting ALS. It begins with supporting life. And in terrain medicine, that begins with the soil.

Who This Book Is For

This book is for you, the person who has just received an ALS diagnosis, or who loves someone who has. It's for the one searching late at night for something, anything, that feels more grounding than a prognosis. It's for the caregiver who feels helpless watching decline and wants to offer support that doesn't feel hollow. It's for the patient who senses that there's more going on than just neuron death and wants to work with the body instead of giving up on it.

You don't need a medical background to understand this book. You don't need to memorize biochemistry or interpret lab results. What you need is willingness. A desire to understand what your body is doing and why. A willingness to listen more closely to what it needs. And the patience to allow healing to come in layers, not all at once.

This isn't a protocol. It's a map. And that map will look different for each person. You don't need to follow every step, or start at the "beginning," or do this perfectly. What you do need is a sense that your body is still capable of responding, and that you can meet it where it is without fear or force.

4

Most importantly: this book is not a promise of a cure. It is a promise of care. It offers a pathway to more stable energy, deeper rest, improved digestion, better emotional regulation, and, most importantly, a renewed sense of dignity and agency in your own healing.

You are not broken. And you're not alone. This book is here to walk beside you, step by step, layer by layer, root by root.

What This Book Does and Doesn't Do

This book offers something different from what you may have seen elsewhere, not a miracle cure or a battle plan, but a step-by-step terrain map designed to restore rhythm, function, and inner coherence. It simplifies complex science into something usable. Something you can begin, right now, without needing a degree or a team of specialists.

It gives you tools, gentle, effective tools, to work with your body instead of against it. Tools to support digestion, calm the immune system, restore sleep, protect energy, and slowly open detox pathways only when the body is ready. It doesn't rush. It doesn't push. It teaches you how to read your own cues and move at a pace that your nervous system can handle.

What this book does not do is promise to fight ALS. That mindset, of war, of attack, of stripping the body down, often makes things worse, not better. This book doesn't push detox before the groundwork is laid. It doesn't tell you there's one protocol, one herb, one diet that fits all. Because there isn't.

This is not a path of domination. It's a path of stewardship.

The terrain-based approach is about learning to listen: to flares, to fatigue, to the body's quiet yes and resounding no. It's about reclaiming a relationship with your own biology, one that is rooted not in fear, but in curiosity, calm, and care.

What this book offers is not control. It's guidance. It's clarity. It's a way forward that honors where you've been and gives shape to where you might go next.

Personal Note on Why This Matters

This book didn't begin in a lab or a clinic. It began to take shape by questions. Honest, uncomfortable, necessary questions about why the body breaks down the way it does, and what it might look like to support, not fight, it. Not to bypass the reality of ALS, but to explore what's still possible inside that reality.

That's where this book came from. Not from the belief that there's one answer or hidden cure, but from the conviction that the terrain matters, and that terrain can change.

I wrote this not just as a researcher or practitioner, but as someone who has stood in the middle of uncertainty and wanted something useful. Something that didn't make wild promises, but also didn't abandon the possibility of improvement. Something that treated the body not as a battlefield, but as an ecosystem capable of healing at its own pace, in its own way, when supported wisely.

This book is the result of that commitment, to offer compassionate, non-dogmatic guidance. To stay rooted in both science and humanity. To make the complex simple without making it shallow.

This is for you, and for the people who stand beside you.

Invitation

As you begin this journey, I invite you to set aside the need to figure everything out at once. You don't have to solve ALS in a day. You don't need to be perfect. You don't need to rush. What you need is space, and support, to begin where you are.

Whether you feel strong and ready, or fragile, confused, and overwhelmed, this book meets you there. It's not asking for more than you can give. It's here to walk alongside you, gently, as you begin to feel your way back into your body. Into rhythm. Into trust.

Let go of the pressure to fight. Let go of the fear that you're already too late. Healing doesn't begin with force. It begins with presence. With listening. With small, steady steps that rebuild the foundation underneath everything else.

That's the heart of this book.

You're not being asked to rebuild the whole tree. You're being invited to nourish the soil. To water the roots. To remember that healing, true healing, doesn't come from the top down. It comes from the ground up.

Let's begin there.

Part 1: A New Map for ALS
Chapter 1: You Are Not Powerless

Reclaiming the Narrative

When someone receives an ALS diagnosis, it's often delivered with a flat, devastating certainty: "There's nothing we can do." In that moment, something far more dangerous than the disease itself can begin to take root, fear, paralysis, and a deep sense of helplessness. This narrative doesn't just communicate facts; it shuts doors. It strips away hope and silences the natural instinct to search, question, and act.

But what if that narrative is incomplete?

ALS is not simply a mysterious, unstoppable disease, it is a signal that the body's internal terrain has been collapsing over time. Like a landscape hit by erosion, pollution, and neglect, the systems that once maintained health begin to break down. And while we may not yet know how to reverse ALS in every case, we do know how to work with terrain.

Reframing ALS in this way does not ignore the seriousness of the condition, it restores agency. It reminds us that biology is not fixed, that the body is responsive, and that there are meaningful actions you can take to shift the trajectory of your health.

You do not need to chase a "cure" to reclaim your quality of life. You do not need to defeat ALS in order to influence it. Even in the face of uncertainty, the possibility of improvement, of stability, clarity, deeper sleep, less pain, more energy, is real. But it begins with a shift in mindset: from resignation to inquiry, from fear to stewardship, from diagnosis to terrain repair.

What Power Really Means in This Context

When people hear the word "power" in the context of healing, they often think of dominance, control, or perfection. But real power, especially when facing a diagnosis like ALS, looks very different. It's quieter, steadier, and more sustainable.

Power, in this context, means having choices. It means being able to shape your daily rhythms in a way that supports healing rather than depletion. It means having access to support, nutritional, emotional, spiritual, environmental, not because you're trying to "beat" the disease, but because your body responds to safety and nourishment more than to force.

Power also means physiological safety. It's not about doing everything right or chasing the perfect protocol. It's about calming the internal stress signals that keep the nervous system stuck in fight, flight, or freeze. Healing begins when the body no longer feels under siege. And even the smallest shifts, deeper sleep, steadier blood sugar, fewer inflammatory foods, can begin to restore that internal safety.

Perhaps most importantly, power means understanding. When you learn what's really happening beneath the surface, when you begin to see ALS not as a random assault but as a breakdown of systems that can be supported and rebuilt, something changes. You stop feeling like a passive victim of biology and start becoming an active steward of your own terrain.

This kind of power isn't loud. It's rooted. And it builds over time.

You Don't Need to Be Perfect, You Need the Right Sequence

One of the biggest traps in any healing journey is the belief that you have to do everything, right now, all at once, and without missteps. But healing, especially in the context of ALS terrain repair, is not about perfection. It's about sequence.

When the body has been under stress for years, even decades, trying to fix everything at once only adds more pressure to an already overwhelmed system. The key is to move in the right order, supporting the body step by step, in a way that builds capacity instead of draining it.

First, we rebuild what's missing: nutrients, energy, rest, rhythm, and safety. Without this foundation, nothing else can hold.

Next, we remove what's harmful, not in a rushed or aggressive way, but thoughtfully. This means reducing inflammatory foods, toxins, and inputs that keep the body in defense mode.

Then we repair what's broken, sealing the gut, supporting the blood-brain barrier, calming the immune system, and restoring mitochondrial function.

Finally, we reconnect what's frozen: the nervous system, the emotional body, the relationships and rhythms that help us feel safe in the world again.

This book is not a to-do list or a one-size-fits-all protocol. It's a layered guide that helps you move through these phases at your own pace, with your own capacities in mind. Healing isn't a sprint, it's a sequencing. And getting the sequence right makes all the difference.

This Book Is Not About False Hope, It's About Real Biology

Hope without grounding can feel hollow, especially when facing a condition like ALS. That's why this book doesn't offer false promises or miracle cures. What it offers instead is a biological framework, a terrain-based approach rooted in how the body actually works.

Terrain medicine is not a magic trick. It's a way of understanding the body as an interconnected system, one that is constantly regenerating, adapting, and responding to its environment. Every day, your body is making decisions, on what to repair, what to protect, what to eliminate, and what to conserve. These decisions are shaped by the inputs it receives: nutrients, toxins, rhythms, thoughts, stressors, and support.

Even in ALS, where it can feel like systems are shutting down, there are still levers you can influence. You can nourish the mitochondria that power your cells. You can calm the immune signals that inflame the nervous system. You can support the gut lining that protects your brain, and the fascia and lymph that carry waste away. These are not abstract ideas, they are biological processes with practical, measurable steps.

This book isn't trying to sell you on blind optimism. It's inviting you to engage with your biology, to work with the body instead of against it. That's not false hope. That's grounded, actionable science. And it's enough to begin.

You Are Not Alone in This

When you're handed a diagnosis like ALS, it can feel like you've been dropped into a vast and silent wilderness. Standard medical paths offer few options. Conversations with doctors may feel cold or rushed. Friends and family might not know what to say, or may quietly step back, unsure of how to help. But despite how isolating this experience can be, you are not alone.

Across the world, thousands of patients, families, and caregivers are quietly finding their way. They are asking new questions, trying new approaches, and witnessing unexpected improvements. They are learning to repair terrain not because they were trained in medicine or biology, but because they refused to accept the idea that nothing could be done.

You do not need to be a doctor to support healing. You do not need to know everything to begin. What you need is curiosity, rhythm, and support. Healing is not a solo act, it is a team effort. And it often begins with something simple yet profound: a shift in perspective.

Instead of asking, "What's wrong with me?" you begin to ask, "What systems have been struggling? What might help them recover?" That shift, toward partnership with the body and collaboration with others, is the first act of reclaiming agency. And in that shift, healing begins.

Chapter 2: The Story We've Been Told

Disempowering narratives dominate: "no cure," "no known cause." These views ignore early clues and deeper biological failures.

The Standard Medical Narrative

From the moment an ALS diagnosis is delivered, patients are often met with a grim and uniform script: "It's progressive. It's untreatable. There's no cure, and we don't know what causes it." These words are repeated across clinics, hospitals, and neurology offices, not as a failure of compassion, but as a reflection of how medicine has been taught to see this disease.

ALS is officially defined as a neurodegenerative condition in which motor neurons, the nerve cells responsible for movement, die off without a known cause. But the way that definition is communicated often strips the moment of all possibility. The diagnosis becomes less a point of inquiry and more a final sentence.

Instead of being rooted in an understanding of what has gone wrong inside the body, the diagnosis is made by exclusion, ruling out other diseases until ALS is what remains. There is no singular test to confirm it. No discovery of root causes. No explanation of what began failing long before symptoms emerged.

What's left is a narrative of helplessness. A story that tells patients and families: There is nothing to explore, nothing to change, nothing to do but wait. And that story, more than the diagnosis itself, can be one of the most damaging parts of the entire journey.

What This Story Leaves Out

The standard medical narrative focuses on what is visible: motor neurons dying, muscles weakening, speech fading. But it rarely asks the deeper question: Why is the nervous system failing in the first place?

What gets missed are the years, or even decades, of signals the body has been quietly sending long before the first neurological symptom appeared. Fatigue that lingers no matter how much you rest. Digestive discomfort that comes and goes, then becomes the norm. Sleep that becomes shallow or fragmented. A background hum of chronic stress or unresolved trauma that never quite lets the system settle.

In most cases, these symptoms are dismissed as unrelated. They're brushed off as aging, anxiety, or coincidence. But they are not separate from the ALS process. They are early terrain warnings, clues that the systems responsible for energy, repair, and resilience have been struggling for a long time.

By ignoring these layers, the standard story not only overlooks what led to the diagnosis, it also blinds us to potential avenues for intervention. The body has been speaking. It's time we started listening.

What Patients Are Rarely Told

In most neurology offices, the conversation about ALS begins and ends with symptoms: when they started, how quickly they're progressing, and what to expect next. But very few patients are ever told what may have been happening beneath the surface, often for years, before those symptoms became visible.

They're not told that mitochondrial dysfunction, the gradual breakdown of the body's energy production systems, can begin silently and go unrecognized for a decade or more. They're not told that the gut lining may have become permeable, allowing toxins and inflammatory signals to seep into circulation, long

14

before any digestive symptom was noticeable. Or that toxic exposures, nutrient depletion, and an overwhelmed immune system may have been slowly eroding the body's resilience over time.

No one mentions how trauma, emotional, physical, or medical, can disrupt nervous system regulation and keep the body stuck in a state of chronic survival. Or how latent infections and subclinical malnutrition can create an invisible but compounding strain on internal systems.

And perhaps most importantly, patients are rarely told that these contributors are not untouchable. There are documented cases of people slowing or stabilizing their symptoms through integrative care, by working with the terrain, not just the diagnosis. These are not miracle stories. They are examples of what becomes possible when we expand the lens and look at the body as a living, dynamic system, one that still responds to care.

Why This Narrative Persists

The story most patients hear about ALS, the one centered on mystery, inevitability, and lack of options, is not just the result of limited knowledge. It's the product of a medical system shaped by its own constraints.

Medical training, for the most part, is built around diagnosing diseases and matching them to pharmaceutical treatments. Doctors are taught to identify symptoms, assign a label, and then follow the standard of care associated with that label. There is little room in this model for systems biology, where multiple body systems are viewed as interconnected. And even less for environmental medicine, where toxins, nutrition, and trauma are taken seriously as drivers of disease.

As a result, ALS research has become narrowly focused: genetics, drug trials, and symptom management. These efforts matter, but they leave out entire layers of terrain collapse that are measurable, modifiable, and clinically relevant. The idea that the terrain might be failing long before neurons die isn't even part of the framework.

And so, "there's no cure" becomes a kind of shorthand. It doesn't always mean "we've tried everything." Often, it means "we haven't explored other models of intervention," or "we don't have the tools, or the language, to talk about what's happening at the systems level."

Add to this the institutional fears of liability and the limitations imposed by insurance billing, and the result is a culture that actively discourages experimentation, even when a patient is willing and informed. Clinicians are often afraid to recommend anything outside the textbook, no matter how logical or low-risk.

This isn't about blaming doctors. It's about recognizing the structural forces that keep the narrative narrow, and choosing to step outside of it when the stakes are too high to wait.

The Cost of This Narrative

The conventional story told around ALS may seem clinical and objective on the surface, but its impact runs deep. When patients are told there's nothing that can be done, it doesn't just shape their understanding of the disease. It shapes their relationship to their own body, their sense of agency, and their willingness to engage.

This narrative robs people of their curiosity, the very instinct that drives us to ask questions, seek patterns, and look for what might still be possible. It strips away momentum in a moment when movement, any movement, is vital. It fosters passivity when what's needed is thoughtful exploration and alignment with the body's deeper signals.

Families, too, are caught in its spell. When they're told there's no path forward, many stop searching. And even well-meaning practitioners may avoid looking into alternative or integrative approaches, not because they're unwilling, but because the medical system has taught them those paths are unscientific or out of bounds.

But the greatest cost may be the delay. Vital systems, like detoxification, nutritional repletion, and neurological rhythm, often go unsupported, precisely when they are most in need. Time that could be spent restoring terrain is lost to waiting, watching, and mourning a decline that might not have been inevitable.

This story, for all its authority, is not neutral. It shapes outcomes. And it's time to choose a different one.

Why We Need a New Story

The goal of a new narrative is not to offer false comfort or magical thinking. It's to offer a map, a way of understanding what's happening beneath the surface, and where meaningful change is still possible.

When we shift the story from "there's nothing to be done" to "here is what can be rebuilt," we return dignity to the patient. We reintroduce direction, rhythm, and momentum. Instead of focusing solely on what is lost, muscle, movement, speech, we begin to focus on what can still be restored: energy production, immune balance, barrier integrity, nervous system regulation.

This new story places terrain collapse, not motor neuron death, at the center of the process. It recognizes that neurons are not failing in isolation. They are responding to an internal environment that has become unstable, inflamed, and under-resourced. And while that environment may be complex, it is not beyond our reach.

This isn't about trading one label for another. It's about replacing a narrative of inevitability with one of stewardship. It's about moving from resignation to engagement. And it's about giving patients and caregivers the most valuable thing they've been denied: a place to begin.

Chapter 3: What ALS Really Is

A collapse in energy, detox, immune balance, and cellular repair. Motor neurons are the visible endpoint, not the root cause.

ALS Is the Final Expression, Not the First Failure

ALS doesn't begin when symptoms appear. It doesn't begin with a tremor in the hand, a stumble while walking, or the slow slurring of words. These visible changes are not the start, they are the culmination.

By the time a diagnosis is made, the body has often been struggling in silence for years. Long before motor neurons begin to fail, there are quieter signals: persistent fatigue, digestive distress that seems minor at first, frequent infections that take longer to clear, or a deep sense of emotional exhaustion that never fully lifts. Often, these are chalked up to stress, aging, or coincidence. But in truth, they are signs of a terrain slowly destabilizing.

Trauma, physical or emotional, can compound the damage. So can chronic exposures to environmental toxins, nutrient depletion, or unresolved infections. These forces don't act all at once, but over time, they wear down the body's resilience and energy reserves.

Motor neurons collapse last, not first. They are the most visible part of the breakdown, and so they capture our attention. But their failure is the final expression of a much longer, deeper process. If we only focus on what is dying, we miss the chance to understand what was silently weakening all along.

This chapter begins where the conventional story ends, by asking not just what is failing, but why.

The Body Breaks Down in Layers

ALS is often described as a neurological disease, but this framing is far too narrow. What we're actually witnessing is the collapse of multiple interconnected systems, not just the death of neurons, but the failure of the body's deeper foundations.

Before motor neurons begin to die, other systems are already unraveling, quietly, gradually, and often unnoticed. The first to falter are the mitochondria, the tiny engines inside our cells responsible for producing energy. When they begin to fail, the body no longer has the fuel it needs for repair, detoxification, or resilience. Fatigue deepens. Recovery slows. Inflammation rises.

Next comes the immune system. What should be a selective, intelligent response becomes chaotic. Inflammation becomes chronic rather than adaptive. Immune cells in the brain, like microglia and mast cells, become overactive. Instead of protecting the nervous system, they begin to harm it.

The gut, one of the body's most important barrier systems, also begins to degrade. The lining becomes permeable, allowing food particles, pathogens, and toxins into the bloodstream. The blood-brain barrier follows, allowing those same triggers to reach the nervous system. Detoxification slows. Lymphatic flow stagnates. Waste accumulates. The fascia tightens, the nerves lose flexibility, and subtle signals between systems begin to distort.

And beneath all of this, the nervous system itself starts to freeze. The vagus nerve, which governs digestion, heart rate, immune signaling, and rest, loses tone. Trauma responses stay stuck in the body. Safety becomes harder to access.

By the time motor neurons fail, these layers have already been under strain for years. ALS is not just a nerve problem, it is a multisystem terrain collapse. And to support healing, we must start where the collapse began.

The Real Drivers Are Often Invisible on Standard Tests

One of the most frustrating realities for patients is that by the time symptoms become undeniable, many conventional tests still come back "normal." It's not uncommon to be told your MRI looks fine, your labs are within range, and your digestive system shows no obvious signs of distress, despite feeling profoundly unwell.

But normal doesn't mean optimal. And standard tests weren't designed to detect the slow, cumulative breakdowns that define terrain collapse.

You can have significant mitochondrial dysfunction, cells struggling to produce energy, without a single abnormality on imaging. You can have a leaky gut and a compromised blood-brain barrier, allowing toxins and immune triggers into circulation, without any GI symptoms at all. And you can be in a state of immune dysregulation, with chronic low-grade inflammation and misfiring immune cells, even if your CBC looks completely unremarkable.

These imbalances live below the surface of standard neurology. They don't show up on the tests most doctors are trained to run, and they don't fit neatly into the definitions most specialists are taught to look for.

So instead of discovering root causes, patients are often handed a label, ALS, and left to navigate a system that doesn't ask what allowed that label to emerge in the first place.

But what standard medicine misses, systems biology can begin to reveal. The real story isn't in the label. It's in the Collapse ≠ Random

There's a common misconception that ALS strikes at random, that it descends out of nowhere, like a bolt of lightning. But when you look more closely at the biology, a different picture emerges, one that is layered, patterned, and far from accidental.

Mitochondria don't simply fail without cause. They degrade under pressure, chronic toxin exposure, nutrient depletion, oxidative stress, infections, and trauma all chip away at their ability to generate energy. Barriers like the gut lining and blood-brain barrier don't spontaneously break down either. They lose integrity slowly, as inflammation smolders, as the terrain becomes undernourished, and as the immune system remains on constant alert.

Chronic inflammation doesn't arise in a vacuum. It builds when the body can no longer resolve immune responses, when detoxification stalls, when microbes overgrow and the vagus nerve stays in freeze mode. And emotional shutdown, the loss of resilience, the retreat into numbness or despair, isn't a personality flaw. It's a physiological survival strategy in response to overwhelming, unresolved stress.

Together, these forces create the conditions in which neurons become vulnerable. ALS is not just about nerve death, it's about the biological stress that leads to that breakdown. It's not a freak event. It's a cascade. And once we recognize the sequence, we can begin to intervene, system by system, layer by layer.

Understanding that collapse follows a pattern doesn't guarantee reversal. But it does offer something just as important: the possibility of direction, logic, and influence in a process once thought to be untouchable.

Why Terrain Matters More Than Labels

A diagnosis can be clarifying. It can give a name to a collection of frightening symptoms and bring a sense of understanding, however limited. But naming the disease, calling it ALS, doesn't fix what made the body vulnerable in the first place. A label may help organize treatment plans or insurance codes, but it doesn't restore balance to the systems that have collapsed.

That's why healing begins not with the label, but with the terrain. The question is not simply "How do we stop neuron death?" but "What broke down in the body that allowed this process to begin?"

When we shift the focus from treating ALS to rebuilding terrain, everything changes. We stop chasing surface symptoms and start tracing the deeper disruptions, energy loss, immune confusion, gut damage, toxic overload, trauma imprint. And instead of searching for a cure in the abstract, we start making practical moves in the present.

This doesn't mean denying the diagnosis. It means refusing to let the diagnosis define your entire path forward. You are not just managing ALS. You are working with your biology, system by system, step by step, to restore the ground it stands on.

Because terrain is where disease begins. And terrain is where healing begins, too.

Chapter 4: Understanding Terrain Collapse

Breakdowns happen in layers: mitochondria, immune dysregulation, gut and barrier damage, fascia, lymph, and vagus nerve freeze. Early symptoms (fatigue, GI issues, sleep trouble) are early warnings.

Collapse Is Not Sudden, It's Sequential

To many patients, ALS feels like it arrives without warning. One day everything seems normal, and the next, something is off, muscles twitching, hands weakening, speech faltering. But in truth, the collapse that leads to ALS is almost never sudden. It unfolds quietly, over years.

Long before the nervous system visibly breaks down, the body begins sending softer signals. Fatigue that doesn't go away with rest. Brain fog that disrupts clarity. Trouble sleeping, even in calm environments. Digestive sensitivities that come and go, then linger. These symptoms are often ignored, minimized, or misdiagnosed, written off as stress, age, or unrelated quirks.

But they are not random. They are early warnings. Each one points to a deeper disturbance in the terrain, a slow unraveling of the systems that keep the body resilient, adaptable, and stable. What may look like separate problems are, in fact, part of a single unfolding process.

Understanding this sequence matters. It helps us see that ALS does not appear from nowhere, and it reminds us that intervention is not limited to late stages. If we can read the signals early, we can begin to support the terrain before the most visible breakdown occurs.

Collapse is not instant. It's a progression. And every point along that path is a chance to act.

Mitochondria: The First to Falter

At the very foundation of every cell in the body are mitochondria, the microscopic power plants that generate the energy needed for life. They produce ATP, the fuel that powers everything from muscle contraction and brain signaling to immune response and tissue repair. Without enough ATP, the body doesn't just slow down, it begins to falter at every level.

In the early stages of terrain collapse, mitochondrial dysfunction is often the first system to go off course. When mitochondria can't keep up, cells don't have the energy to detoxify, defend, or repair themselves. The result is a cascade of low energy, persistent fatigue, poor recovery from stress or illness, and mounting oxidative damage inside tissues.

This dysfunction rarely appears out of nowhere. It's typically triggered by chronic, cumulative stressors that wear the mitochondria down over time. Environmental toxins, such as heavy metals, mold toxins, and glyphosate, are common culprits. So are viral infections and stealth pathogens that hide beneath the radar of standard tests, quietly exhausting the body's reserves. Add to that nutrient deficiencies, poor sleep, and long-term emotional stress, and the terrain begins to slip into an energy deficit.

Once this energy crisis sets in, other systems follow. Detoxification slows. Inflammation rises. The immune system becomes dysregulated. And though the visible symptoms may still be years away, the groundwork for collapse has already begun.

To support healing, we must return to this foundational layer. Because without restoring cellular energy, no other repair can hold.

Immune System: From Balance to Chaos

A healthy immune system is not just aggressive, it's intelligent. Its job isn't simply to attack, but to discern. It should recognize what belongs, respond swiftly to true threats, and then stand down when safety is restored. But in terrain collapse, that balance begins to break.

One of the first signs of this shift is in the brain. Microglia, the immune cells that patrol the nervous system, become overactive. What should be a calm, protective force turns hyper-vigilant. These cells begin reacting to even minor stimuli as if they're dangerous, releasing inflammatory compounds that damage nearby neurons and tissue.

Mast cells, another branch of the immune system, also lose their rhythm. Instead of releasing histamine and signaling molecules when truly needed, they begin to fire chronically. This leads to an ongoing flood of inflammatory signals that affects not just the brain, but the gut, skin, lungs, and more.

At the heart of this process is a feedback loop of stress. Cytokines, chemical messengers of the immune system, amplify inflammation, disrupt sleep, interfere with digestion, and perpetuate a sense of internal unease. The nervous system becomes agitated. The body stays on high alert. And healing, which depends on calm and safety, becomes increasingly difficult.

This isn't just an immune system that's confused. It's one that has lost its ability to shift gears. And until we help it return to balance, inflammation will continue smoldering, especially in the delicate tissues of the nervous system.

Gut, Brain, and Barrier Breakdown

The body is protected by more than just skin. Deep inside, there are internal barriers that keep us safe at the cellular level, gatekeepers that decide what stays out and what passes through. Two of the most critical are the gut lining and the blood-brain barrier. When they're intact, they maintain order. When they break down, chaos follows.

In terrain collapse, the gut lining is often one of the first barriers to weaken. This condition, commonly referred to as "leaky gut", allows undigested food particles, toxins, and bacterial fragments to slip into the bloodstream. These intruders aren't supposed to be there, and their presence sets off immune alarms that drive widespread inflammation.

As this gut barrier falters, a similar breakdown often begins in the brain. The blood-brain barrier (BBB), which normally keeps the brain protected from circulating toxins and immune triggers, becomes porous. Once it's compromised, substances that should never reach the brain can pass through, fueling neuroinflammation and disturbing neural function.

These barrier failures don't happen randomly. They're the result of sustained stress on the terrain. Poor nutrition weakens the structural integrity of both the gut and brain linings. A high toxic burden, pesticides, heavy metals, mold, erodes resilience further. Emotional trauma, especially when unprocessed, keeps the nervous system in a constant state of tension. And underlying it all, mitochondrial depletion robs these tissues of the energy they need to repair and protect themselves.

When these barriers fall, the body's internal world becomes exposed, disordered, and inflamed. But with the right support, even damaged barriers can begin to seal again.

Symptoms Are Signals, Not Surprises

We're taught to minimize symptoms. To push through fatigue. To blame food reactions on age or stress. To dismiss brain fog, poor sleep, skin irritation, or anxiety as just "modern life." But these early symptoms aren't random. They're the body waving a flag, sometimes quietly, sometimes urgently, saying, "The terrain is struggling."

Feeling "just tired" every afternoon isn't a personality flaw or a caffeine deficiency. It's often a sign of mitochondrial overload, blood sugar instability, or chronic inflammation. Becoming "just sensitive to certain foods" is rarely about pickiness, it's a reflection of increased gut permeability, immune overactivation, or an overloaded detox system.

Sleep troubles, histamine reactions, bloating, brain fog, shortness of breath, and nerve twitching are not isolated issues. They are expressions of a bigger pattern: the breakdown of balance in the body's terrain.

The good news? These signals are useful. They give us insight, feedback, and direction. When we learn to listen, without fear, without rushing to suppress them, we start to map where the system is overwhelmed and what it's asking for. In this model, symptoms are not surprises. They are clues. And when interpreted with care, they point the way toward repair.

Chapter 5: What Doctors Miss

Fragmented care and diagnostic silos ignore root cause terrain issues. ALS diagnosis is made by exclusion, not explanation. You don't have time to wait for the system to catch up.

Medicine Is Fragmented Into Silos

In conventional medicine, the body is divided into compartments. If your nerves are affected, you see a neurologist. If your digestion is off, you're sent to a gastroenterologist. If your immune system is dysregulated, that's an immunologist's domain. Struggling with mood, sleep, or cognition? That's for psychiatry.

This fragmented approach may seem organized, but it often misses the forest for the trees, especially in complex conditions like ALS. Because ALS affects motor neurons, it's typically treated as a purely neurological disease. Yet mounting evidence shows that people with ALS also exhibit signs of gut permeability, immune overactivation, mitochondrial dysfunction, heavy metal accumulation, and limbic system dysregulation.

When each specialist only examines their designated part of the body, the broader terrain collapse is often overlooked. The result is a scattered view of what is, in truth, a deeply interconnected system in crisis.

True healing begins when we stop chasing symptoms in isolation and start seeing the terrain as a whole. ALS doesn't live in just one part of the body, and neither does the path to recovery.

ALS Diagnosis Is Based on Elimination

Unlike infections or genetic disorders that can be confirmed by a single test, ALS is diagnosed by exclusion. That means doctors arrive at the diagnosis not by discovering a clear cause, but by ruling everything else out.

Most people with ALS spend years experiencing unexplained symptoms long before a diagnosis is ever mentioned. It often begins with subtle fatigue, gut issues, food sensitivities, anxiety, or muscle twitching. These early clues are frequently dismissed, minimized, or misattributed, especially when basic labs return "within normal range."

Imaging studies like MRIs or nerve conduction tests (EMG) are usually ordered late in the process, often only after functional decline becomes visible. Once other neurological diseases like multiple sclerosis or myasthenia gravis are excluded, the label of ALS is given. But the question of why, why the body began to break down in the first place, is rarely pursued.

This absence of root-cause inquiry leaves patients without a framework for healing. But that's where a terrain-based model begins: by asking what terrain conditions allowed the collapse, and how to rebuild from the ground up.

Root-Cause Testing Is Rarely Done

By the time someone is diagnosed with ALS, the underlying terrain has often been breaking down for years. But in most cases, the systems that failed first are never investigated at all.

Patients are almost never tested for mitochondrial health, the energy factories that power every cell, including neurons. Environmental toxicants like mold, mercury, aluminum, or glyphosate aren't measured, even though they are known to impair nerve function and immune regulation. Gut permeability and microbiome imbalances, which can drive inflammation throughout the brain and body, are rarely considered.

Likewise, few clinicians explore the patient's immune terrain:

whether chronic viral infections like EBV or HHV-6 are active, or whether the innate immune system is stuck in a hypervigilant loop. And nearly no one asks how early life trauma, grief, or chronic stress might have impacted the nervous system's long-term resilience.

By the time motor neurons begin to visibly degenerate, these deeper systems have often been collapsing silently for years. But without looking there, conventional medicine concludes that ALS is simply "idiopathic", meaning, without a known cause. A terrain model offers a different view: one that sees the body's distress signals long before the final breakdown.

Why the System Isn't Built for Terrain Thinking

The conventional medical system is designed to save lives in crisis, not to rebuild health over time. Medical education emphasizes acute care, diagnostic algorithms, and risk management. Doctors are trained to look for patterns that match known diseases and to intervene quickly when those patterns escalate into emergencies.

But terrain collapse, the slow unraveling of the body's self-regulating systems, is neither fast nor straightforward. It doesn't fit into a 15-minute appointment slot. It doesn't trigger standard lab abnormalities early on. And it doesn't respond well to single-target medications.

By the time ALS enters the picture, patients have already passed through years of subclinical decline. Yet the diagnosis is often treated as a final answer, not a red flag pointing to deeper causes. Once the ALS label is applied, the investigation stops. Support becomes focused on symptom management, assistive devices, and end-of-life planning.

In this model, the diagnosis becomes a wall. In terrain medicine, it becomes a doorway.

Patients Are Left in Limbo

For many individuals diagnosed with ALS, the conversation ends before it ever truly begins. After months or even years of unexplained symptoms, vague reassurances, and dismissals, they're finally handed a label, only to be told there's no cure, no treatment that slows progression meaningfully, and no known cause.

The message is often delivered with finality:
"It's probably genetic."
"Sometimes these things just happen."
"All we can do now is support your quality of life."

This framing does more than disappoint, it shuts down curiosity. It discourages both patients and families from seeking further answers, and it subtly warns them not to trust anything outside of conventional consensus. Exploring "unproven" therapies or asking about alternative strategies is often met with skepticism, or even quiet disapproval.

But when you're told there is nothing to be done, you are also being told not to look. Not to question. Not to investigate the slow terrain breakdown that led to this point.

This leaves many patients suspended in a kind of medical limbo: dismissed by one system, but not yet empowered by another. That's where this book steps in, not to replace medical care, but to reopen the door to biological possibility. To show that the body's story didn't begin with ALS, and it doesn't have to end with it either.

You Don't Have Time to Wait

There's a growing movement within medicine that recognizes the importance of systems biology, functional testing, and root-cause healing. But it's not yet the standard of care, and for someone facing an ALS diagnosis, waiting for the system to catch up simply isn't an option.

The good news is: you don't have to wait.

Right now, you can begin taking steps that support the systems most commonly in distress long before motor neuron loss becomes visible. You can begin nourishing your mitochondria, the tiny energy producers that power every cell in your brain, muscles, and nerves. You can start sealing and healing your gut, calming the immune system, and improving nutrient absorption. You can remove toxicants that overload your detox and lymphatic pathways, like fluoride, aluminum, mold, or harmful seed oils. You can gently retrain your nervous system from a state of chronic alarm into one of regulation and resilience.

You don't need a perfect plan. You need momentum. Small steps, when aimed in the right direction, can shift the trajectory of your terrain. And while mainstream research continues to search for pharmaceutical breakthroughs, you can begin rebuilding the foundations your body needs to heal.

Every day counts. Every meal, every breath, every choice that reduces burden or adds nourishment matters. The earlier you begin supporting your terrain, the more opportunity you create for the body to respond.

Part 2: Rebuilding the Terrain

Chapter 6: Replete Before You Detox

The terrain is starved, nutritionally, energetically, emotionally. Repletion is the foundation: minerals, fats, protein, electrolytes, B vitamins. Key signs of readiness: deeper sleep, steadier energy, regular elimination.

ALS Terrain Is Starved, Not Just Toxic

In many chronic illness protocols, the first step is often detox, clearing out heavy metals, pathogens, or environmental chemicals believed to be disrupting the system. But in ALS, starting with detox is not only ineffective, it can be dangerous.

That's because the ALS terrain isn't just toxic. It's profoundly starved.

Underneath the surface, the body is already depleted. Mitochondria, the microscopic engines that produce ATP, your cellular energy currency, are underperforming. Nutrient reserves are low, often due to gut dysfunction, poor absorption, long-standing food restrictions, or decades of low-grade inflammation. Essential minerals like magnesium, zinc, and potassium may be deficient. Fat-soluble vitamins (like A, D, E, and K2) that support nerve health are frequently underutilized or missing altogether.

At the same time, the terrain is overloaded with stress. This includes not just emotional trauma, but also metabolic strain, oxidative damage, and the physical toll of disrupted sleep, blood sugar swings, and unresolved inflammation.

In this fragile state, jumping straight into detoxification can overwhelm an already struggling system. Mobilizing toxins before the body has the resources to excrete them properly can lead to flare-ups, regressions, or even further degeneration. That's why a terrain-based approach to ALS begins with repletion, not removal. We feed the system first. We rebuild its strength. Only then can it safely begin the work of letting go.

What Repletion Means

Repletion isn't just about taking a multivitamin and hoping for the best. It's a full-body commitment to rebuilding the raw materials your cells need to repair, regulate, and regenerate. In terrain medicine, repletion is the foundation, what you do before you begin detoxing, before pushing therapies, and before addressing deeper layers of dysfunction.

Think of it like tending to depleted soil. You wouldn't start ripping out weeds from dry, barren ground, you'd water it first. Add minerals. Introduce compost. Create an environment where new life could actually take hold. The same principle applies here. Before asking your body to heal, you must give it what it needs to feel nourished, stable, and safe.

This includes:

Macronutrients: Adequate high-quality protein and healthy fats are essential. They provide the structural building blocks for muscle repair, neurotransmitter production, and cellular membranes. In ALS, muscle breakdown and metabolic stress can quickly outpace intake if these needs aren't met.

Micronutrients: Vitamins and minerals like magnesium, zinc, B12, selenium, and CoQ10 serve as enzyme cofactors for mitochondrial energy production and nerve conduction. Deficiencies are common in ALS terrain and must be corrected for healing to begin.

Electrolytes: Sodium, potassium, magnesium, calcium, chloride, and other trace minerals work together to regulate hydration, nerve conduction, and muscle function. These charged minerals are the foundation of electrical stability in the body. When the terrain is inflamed, depleted, or under stress, electrolytes are quickly lost, yet they are essential for restoring balance, energy, and communication between cells.

Rest and Rhythm: True repletion isn't just nutritional. The body also needs cues of safety. Sleep, gentle daily rhythm, breath work, and nervous system down-regulation allow the healing state (the parasympathetic mode) to take over. Without it, repair stalls no matter what you feed the body.

Repletion is the signal to your terrain that it's time to rebuild. And only when the body feels resourced, physically and neurologically, can the deeper healing work begin.

Key Nutrients for Mitochondria, Nerves, and Terrain Integrity

When the terrain is in collapse, the nervous system isn't the only part suffering, your mitochondria, immune system, detox pathways, and structural tissues are all struggling to stay functional. But without the right inputs, these systems can't repair themselves. That's where strategic repletion comes in.

Below are some of the most important nutrients for people with ALS and similar neurodegenerative terrain patterns. These nutrients don't just "support health" in a general way, they actively participate in restoring the body's energy flow, calming inflammation, and protecting nerve structure at the cellular level.

Magnesium (glycinate or malate forms)

Magnesium is involved in over 300 enzymatic reactions, including those needed to create ATP, the fuel mitochondria produce. It also calms the nervous system, reduces muscle cramping, aids bowel movements, and helps the body process toxins. Many people with ALS are magnesium-deficient, especially if they're under chronic stress or on medications that deplete it.

Potassium
Potassium doesn't get enough attention, but it's essential for nerve signaling, adrenal stability, and intracellular hydration. It helps maintain calm and steady communication between nerves and muscles. In ALS terrain, low potassium can worsen fatigue, cramps, and blood pressure instability.

B-Vitamins (especially B1, B6, B12, and folate)
These vitamins fuel critical mitochondrial enzymes, help repair nerve sheaths, and assist in detoxifying harmful compounds like homocysteine. Low B12 and B1 are common in neurodegeneration and can mimic or worsen ALS symptoms if left unaddressed.

Vitamin D + K2
These fat-soluble vitamins work together to regulate immune function, calcium distribution, and even mitochondrial biogenesis (the creation of new mitochondria). Vitamin D alone isn't enough, K2 helps direct calcium into bones and out of soft tissues, preventing nerve-damaging calcification.

Omega-3 Fatty Acids (EPA and DHA)
Found in fish oil or algae oil, these powerful anti-inflammatory fats help protect brain and nerve tissue, rebuild damaged membranes, and modulate immune activity. They're essential in any terrain restoration plan focused on neuroprotection.

Low-Dose Lithium (nutritional microdose, not psychiatric

dose)

Trace amounts of lithium orotate have been shown to support mitochondrial integrity, calm mood instability, and promote nerve growth factor. This is very different from prescription lithium carbonate, used in much higher doses for bipolar disorder, and may offer neuroprotective benefits at safe microdose levels.

Chlorophyll (and Chlorophyllin)

While best known for its role in plants, chlorophyll plays a surprising role in human mitochondrial health. It enhances mitochondrial ATP production by acting as a light-activated electron donor, essentially helping mitochondria produce more energy when exposed to red and near-infrared light. Chlorophyll also binds to toxic compounds and facilitates their removal, reducing the burden on cellular detox pathways. Some forms, like chlorophyllin, have been shown to protect mitochondrial membranes from oxidative damage and may help stabilize energy production in terrain-collapse states like ALS.

These nutrients form the backbone of a terrain-aware repletion strategy. Without them, the body remains stuck in survival mode. With them, healing becomes biologically possible.

Food-Based Repletion Strategies

Supplements can play an important therapeutic role, especially when digestion is impaired or specific deficiencies are urgent. But long-term terrain repair depends on nutrient-dense, whole foods. Food is not just fuel; it's information. It tells your body what kind of environment it's living in: one of depletion, or one of restoration.

In ALS and related terrain collapse, the body is starved not just for calories, but for deep nourishment. The goal is to consistently feed the mitochondria, calm the immune system, support detox pathways, and rebuild tissues with ingredients the body recognizes and can absorb.

Some of the most powerful repletion comes from:

Proteins
Healing requires complete proteins, especially those rich in amino acids like glycine, glutamine, and proline. Foods like grass-fed liver, pastured meats, collagen-rich bone broth, whole eggs, and sardines with bonesoffer the nutrients needed for muscle repair, neurotransmitter formation, and gut lining integrity.

Fats
Healthy fats are not just tolerated, they are essential in ALS terrain. Fats like grass-fed ghee, extra virgin olive oil, virgin coconut oil, and egg yolks provide cholesterol (critical for myelin sheaths), fat-soluble vitamins, and anti-inflammatory support. They also help stabilize blood sugar and provide dense, usable energy.

Mineral-Rich Foods
Minerals run the body's electrical system. Rebuilding electrolyte and cofactor status requires everyday sources like pumpkin seeds (zinc and magnesium), blackstrap molasses (iron, potassium, and calcium), and cooked dark leafy greens (a broad spectrum of trace minerals and chlorophyll).

Green Superfood Powders
While not a replacement for whole fruits and vegetables, green powders are concentrated way to boost daily nutrient density without extra calories or digestive burden. These blends often contain powdered spinach, kale, wheatgrass, chlorella, spirulina, and other deeply pigmented greens, each packed with chlorophyll, magnesium, enzymes, and trace minerals. They support mitochondrial health, detoxification, and pH balance, while

delivering plant-based antioxidants in an easy-to-absorb form. Add scoops to water, smoothies, or coconut water can significantly upgrade the terrain's message: nourishment is here, and healing can begin.

Bulk Herbs as Nutritive Tonics

Some herbs aren't just medicine, they're food. Nettle leaf, oatstraw, hibiscus, and dandelion leaf are gentle, nourishing plants that support the kidneys, blood, lymph, and adrenal system. These herbs can be brewed daily into teas or infusions that hydrate while delivering minerals and phytonutrients in a highly absorbable form.

Together, these foods send a clear message to the terrain: you are safe, supported, and resourced enough to begin healing.

Supplement-Based Repletion: What to Take and Why

Minerals and Electrolytes:

Magnesium (glycinate or malate)

> Calms the nervous system, supports ATP production, eases muscle tension, and promotes elimination.

> Recommended: Pure Encapsulations Magnesium (Glycinate or Malate).

Potassium (citrate or gluconate)

> Essential for nerve-muscle signaling, hydration, adrenal function, and mitochondrial activity.

> Recommended: Integrative Therapeutics Potassium Citrate (if using under supervision).

Trace minerals

> Fill silent deficiencies that impair detox, nerve signaling, and

repair.

Recommended: Pure Encapsulations Mineral 650 or Quinton Isotonic (for gentle, marine-based repletion).

B-Vitamins and Methylation Cofactors

Thiamine (B1 as benfotiamine or allithiamine)

Vital for mitochondrial enzymes, neuroprotection, and energy regulation.

Recommended: Integrative Therapeutics Benfotiamine.

B6 (P5P), B12 (methylcobalamin or hydroxycobalamin), Folate (methylfolate or folinic acid)

Support nerve sheath repair, neurotransmitter balance, and homocysteine clearance.

Recommended: Pure Encapsulations B-Complex Plus or Homocysteine Factors.

Fat-Soluble Vitamins

Vitamin D3 with K2 (MK-7)

Modulates immune response, calcium handling, and supports mitochondrial biogenesis.

Recommended: Pure Encapsulations D3 with K2.

Vitamin A (retinyl palmitate)

Promotes immune defense, gut lining integrity, and skin/ nerve repair.

Recommended: Integrative Therapeutics Vitamin A.

Vitamin E (mixed tocopherols and tocotrienols)

Stabilizes membranes and protects against oxidative stress.

Recommended: Pure Encapsulations Gamma E Mixed Tocopherols.

Mitochondrial and Nerve Regeneration

CoQ10 (as ubiquinol)

Critical for ATP production, antioxidant recycling, and cell survival.

Recommended: Pure Encapsulations Ubiquinol-QH 200 mg. Pure encapsualtions also has a CoQ10 500mg but it gets costly.

Acetyl-L-Carnitine

Enhances fatty acid transport into mitochondria and supports nerve regeneration.

Recommended: Douglas Labs Acetyl L-Carnitine.

Alpha-lipoic acid (R-ALA form)

Recharges other antioxidants, reduces inflammation, and improves insulin sensitivity.

Recommended: Pure Encapsulations Alpha Lipoic Acid.

Omega-3 and Phospholipid Support

EPA/DHA (from fish oil or algae)

Reduce neuroinflammation, support brain membrane repair, and stabilize mood.

Recommended: Pure Encapsulations EPA/DHA Essentials.

Phosphatidylcholine

Supports bile flow, mitochondrial membranes, and nerve conduction.

Recommended: Integrative Therapeutics Phosphatidylcholine.

Terrain Modulators and Mood Resilience

Low-dose lithium (as lithium orotate)

Supports neuroprotection, mitochondrial integrity, and emotional stability.

Recommended: Pure Encapsulations Lithium (Orotate) 5 mg.

Magnesium L-threonate

Specifically targets the brain to enhance cognitive clarity and nervous system tone.

Recommended: Integrative Therapeutics Magtein.

Foundational Multinutrient Support

High-potency multivitamin with bioavailable forms

Covers nutritional bases while avoiding unnecessary fillers or synthetic additives. This can replace a good portion of the individual supplements listed above.

Recommended: Pure Encapsulations Nutrient 950 (with or without iron, depending on labs).

Emotional and Circadian Repletion

Repletion isn't just physical. Healing the terrain also requires restoring rhythm, both in the body's circadian cycles and in the emotional nervous system. These two systems are deeply connected: how you sleep, how you feel, and how safe your body perceives its environment directly affect your ability to detox, digest, repair, and regenerate.

Sleep is not just rest, it's a daily biological reset. During deep sleep, the brain clears toxins, the immune system recalibrates, and mitochondria repair themselves. But quality sleep only happens when your circadian rhythm is intact. That rhythm is set by light exposure, meal timing, and calming evening routines, not just a dark room and a white noise machine.

At the same time, emotional depletion is often overlooked in clinical settings. Living with ALS, or even just navigating unexplained symptoms before diagnosis, can create chronic stress, fear, grief, and overwhelm. Trauma doesn't have to mean one dramatic event. It can mean years of subtle dysregulation, internalized pressure, or unprocessed emotion. These states wear down the nervous system's ability to shift into healing mode.

To replenish this layer of the terrain, focus on:

Connection: With others, with nature, with purpose. Isolation fuels inflammation; connection rebuilds coherence.

Sunlight: Especially in the morning. Natural light on the eyes and skin anchors your circadian clock and lifts mood by regulating melatonin and serotonin.

Rhythmic activities: Simple, calming rituals like walking, swimming, slow cooking, gentle rocking, or gardening help regulate the vagus nerve and re-establish internal safety.

Vagal support: Breathwork, humming, chanting, nature immersion, and cold exposure gently stimulate the vagus nerve, shifting the body into parasympathetic (rest-and-digest) mode where real healing begins.

When the emotional terrain is nourished, and the body is living in rhythm instead of reaction, healing isn't just possible. It becomes inevitable.

How to Know You're Ready for Detox

In terrain-based healing, detox is not the first step, it's the reward for successful repletion. Before you ask your body to mobilize and release stored toxins, you must be sure it has the strength, energy, and drainage capacity to do so safely. Otherwise, detox becomes damage.

But how do you know when your system is ready?

The signs are subtle but clear. After weeks or months of consistent repletion, through nourishing foods, essential nutrients, hydration, sleep, and nervous system safety, the terrain starts to shift. Energy begins to stabilize. Digestion improves. The whole system starts to move out of survival mode and into repair mode.

Key signals that you're ready to introduce gentle detox strategies include:

Steadier energy throughout the day
You no longer crash after meals or rely on stimulants to get through the morning. There's a baseline steadiness that wasn't there before.

Regular bowel movements and improved elimination
Detox can't work if toxins can't exit. Daily, formed bowel movements signal that the liver, gallbladder, and colon are cooperating, critical for safe detoxification.

Warmer hands and feet, improved circulation
When blood flow returns to the periphery, it's a sign the body is shifting out of fight-or-freeze mode. Detox requires movement, of blood, lymph, and bile, and warmth supports that.

Deeper, more restorative sleep
Sleep is when detoxification ramps up, especially in the brain (via the glymphatic system). If you're falling asleep more easily and waking with less fog, your nervous system is likely ready.

Calmer, more responsive emotional tone
You may notice fewer anxiety spikes, shorter recovery from stress, and greater resilience in your reactions. This emotional flexibility reflects nervous system safety, a prerequisite for terrain detox work.

When these signs are present, your body is telling you: "I'm resourced enough to let go." That's when detox becomes not just safer, but more effective.

Chapter 7: IgG Food Sensitivities and Calming the Gut/Immune System

The Importance of Gut Health Before Detoxification

Before you can begin clearing toxins from the body, your gut needs to be ready to handle the traffic. The gastrointestinal tract is not just a digestive organ, it's one of your body's most important defense systems. It acts as a selective barrier, deciding what enters your bloodstream and what gets safely excreted. When that barrier is compromised, the entire detox process becomes riskier.

In ALS terrain, the gut is often inflamed, fragile, or underperforming. Years of stress, poor absorption, food sensitivities, infections, or medications can weaken the tight junctions in the intestinal lining. This condition, commonly called "leaky gut," allows partially digested food particles, bacterial fragments, and even environmental toxins to slip into systemic circulation. Once inside, they provoke immune alarm bells, increase inflammation, and overwhelm the liver and lymphatic systems that are already under strain.

At the same time, a dysfunctional gut struggles to absorb the very nutrients the body needs for healing, like magnesium, zinc, B vitamins, and amino acids. Without these, you can't properly produce bile, activate detox enzymes, or fuel your mitochondria. This is why jumping straight into detoxification, without first calming and sealing the gut, can backfire. It may lead to new symptoms, worsen inflammation, or stir up toxins that the body can't safely process or eliminate.

By focusing on gut repair first, you create a stable foundation. A strong gut lining filters out harmful substances, keeps immune activation in check, and helps the body get full use of every meal and supplement. Only once that system is calm, nourished, and moving well should detox begin.

Detox is not about force, it's about flow. And the gut is where that flow starts.

IgG Food Sensitivity Testing as an Immune Map, Not a Banned Foods List

This section is intentionally more detailed than others, because few topics in terrain healing are as misunderstood, controversial, or clinically important as IgG food sensitivity testing. While some practitioners dismiss these panels outright, that dismissal often stems from a misunderstanding of what IgG testing actually reveals. In a system where the gut is leaking, the immune system is overactive, and the terrain is inflamed, IgG reactivity isn't meaningless noise, it's a map of where tolerance has broken down.

Understanding and correctly interpreting IgG patterns can be one of the most powerful ways to calm the immune system, reduce symptoms, and begin healing the gut. This depth is necessary to correct common myths, expose flaws in mainstream critiques, and equip you with the clarity to use this tool strategically, not fearfully or blindly. What follows isn't just theory, it's a key to unlocking immune resilience.

The Terrain-Based Purpose of IgG Food Sensitivity Testing

In terrain medicine, every symptom is a signal, not just of what is broken, but of what is burdened. This is especially true when it comes to food sensitivity testing, which is often misunderstood or misapplied in both conventional and alternative settings. IgG-based food panels, when properly ordered and interpreted, offer insight not into "good" or "bad" foods, but into the state of immune tolerance and barrier function across the entire terrain.

The immune system's job is not only to defend against pathogens but also to maintain a memory of what it has been exposed to. In a healthy, intact terrain, foods pass through the gastrointestinal tract, are digested and absorbed efficiently, and are met with a calm, regulated immune response. This is known as oral tolerance, a state in which the immune system recognizes common food antigens as safe. But in terrain collapse, particularly in cases of ALS, neuroinflammation, or autoimmune activation, this tolerance is often broken.

When the gut barrier is compromised, foods are no longer fully digested before fragments cross into the bloodstream. This can occur because of tight junction breakdown, microbial imbalances, parasitic activity, or even translocation from a stagnant lymphatic system. Once these food particles are in circulation, the immune system flags them, often not with the acute, histamine-driven IgE response of a classic allergy, but with IgG antibodies, which mark ongoing or frequent exposure in the context of immune stress.

Importantly, this tagging is not a declaration that the food is toxic. It's a signal that the immune system is overloaded, dysregulated, or confused, especially in the context of chronic exposure to an antigen that should be benign. IgG results, therefore, reflect antigenic load under immune strain. It is not the food's fault, but the terrain's filtration system is failing.

In ALS and related neurodegenerative conditions, this filtration failure isn't limited to the gut. It can include the blood-brain barrier, glymphatic system, and mesenteric lymphatics, all of which rely on clean, regulated immune signaling to prevent nervous system flare-ups. When the gut fails to filter properly, foods that have always been part of the diet suddenly become immunological stressors, provoking not just digestive discomfort but brain fog, fatigue, pain, and systemic inflammation.

This is why IgG panels should be treated as terrain maps, not food lists. They show you where the immune system is encountering friction, where communication has broken down, where tolerance has eroded, and where metabolic congestion is backing up. They do not tell you what foods are "bad." They tell you what foods are being improperly flagged due to immune confusion.

When read in context, not isolation, IgG results can help reveal which exposures are overwhelming an already fragile terrain. And more importantly, they can show where you might relieve some of that burden temporarily, allowing the filtration systems to reset, immune tolerance to rebuild, and food to return to its rightful place as nourishment, not threat.

What IgG Results Really Reflect (And Why They Can Matter Deeply)

To understand the value of IgG food sensitivity testing, you first have to understand what the results actually represent, and what they don't. Unlike IgE, which reflects an acute allergic response that can trigger hives, swelling, or anaphylaxis, IgG antibodies signal chronic exposure and immune recognition over time. They're not reacting to danger per se, they're reacting to familiarity in a terrain under duress.

But not all IgG is created equal. The body produces different subclasses of IgG (IgG1, IgG2, IgG3, and IgG4), and each plays a distinct role in immune signaling. IgG1 and IgG3 tend to be associated with pro-inflammatory responses, the kind that suggest the immune system is agitated and in a state of defense. IgG4, on the other hand, is often interpreted as a marker of tolerance-building, the immune system saying, "I've seen this before, I'm adjusting." Unfortunately, most commercial IgG tests don't differentiate between these subclasses unless you use specialized panels. That makes it even more critical to interpret any elevations through the lens of the patient's immune status, not just the lab's reference range.

Elevated IgG levels against food antigens are not random. They often point to repeated exposure to food particles that have breached the gut lining, a condition commonly referred to as "leaky gut," but more accurately understood as intestinal hyperpermeability. When the mucosal barrier is compromised, large food proteins cross into the bloodstream before they are fully digested. The immune system flags these proteins as potential threats, especially if the terrain is inflamed, toxic, or overloaded. This is why people with severe terrain collapse often show dozens of IgG elevations on a single panel, it's not that all these foods are inherently problematic, it's that the gut is leaking everything into circulation, and the immune system is in a state of alert.

But permeability is not the only driver of IgG reactivity. In some individuals, the immune system has been primed in much deeper ways. Adjuvant exposure from injections, especially aluminum or synthetic emulsifiers used in vaccines, can skew immune surveillance and break tolerance in otherwise benign antigens. This may lead to cross-reactivity, where the immune system confuses a food protein for something more dangerous because of a previous contamination event. Similarly, chronic parasite or viral activation, such as Epstein-Barr virus, Lyme co-infections, or chronic EBV reactivation, can dysregulate the immune response to ingested proteins, creating false danger signalsand collapsing the capacity for tolerance.

In these cases, we are not just looking at "leaky gut." We are looking at a terrain-wide loss of tolerance, one that affects the gut, the nervous system, and the immune blueprint itself. This is why IgG testing can be so powerful: it doesn't just tell you what you're eating. It tells you how your immune system is interpreting your world, through the lens of trauma, overload, infection, and broken filtration.

Importantly, when a true oral intolerance is identified, where a food has become so immunologically charged that it creates systemic symptoms like brain fog, fatigue, pain, or mood instability, removing that food can trigger profound relief. Often, within a matter of days or weeks, the terrain begins to quiet down. What's more, once the primary immune irritants are removed, many of the smaller, less intense IgG reactions begin to resolve on their own. This is not because the test was wrong. It's because removing immune friction allows healing to begin, and with healing comes the return of tolerance.

The key is recognizing that IgG testing doesn't label foods as "bad." It shows you where your immune system is having to work too hard, where it's confused, and where it's overwhelmed. In terrain medicine, that's exactly the kind of intelligence we're looking for, not a list of forbidden foods, but a roadmap to relief.

Why IgG Panels Are Dismissed, And Why That Argument Fails

In the conventional allergy world, IgG testing is often written off entirely. Most allergists and academic critics dismiss these panels because they don't align with the strict IgE model of allergy. According to this framework, only rapid-onset, histamine-mediated reactions, rashes, hives, anaphylaxis, are considered medically valid. Anything slower, subtler, or more systemic is labeled anecdotal or irrelevant. IgG, in this view, is dismissed as simply a marker of exposure, not of intolerance.

But this narrow model completely ignores what terrain-based medicine is observing in real time. In people with autoimmune disease, chronic infection, mast cell dysregulation, or neurodegenerative terrain like ALS, IgG elevations aren't just benign evidence of exposure, they're indicators of a collapsed tolerance system. When the gut is leaky, the immune system is overwhelmed, and filtration systems like the lymphatics and blood-brain barrier are under strain, IgG responses become a reflection of real friction, not just memory.

What most of the mainstream critiques fail to account for is the context in which IgG reactivity becomes pathological. Studies often attempt to invalidate these panels by testing them in healthy individuals with intact barrier systems, normal immune regulation, and no ongoing inflammatory load. Of course they find little correlation with symptoms, because the test isn't meant for people with intact terrain. IgG food reactivity is not a useful diagnostic tool for the general population, it is a map of immune burden in those whose terrain is already compromised.

Even many integrative or functional practitioners fall short, either by over-interpreting every IgG elevation as a banned food or by dismissing the test entirely due to bad experiences with low-quality labs. And that's part of the problem too: many IgG tests are not good tests. Cheap panels often use non-standardized food antigens, have poor quality control, don't measure IgG subclasses, and report vague, non-reproducible results. Worse, many of them don't explain their methodology at all. This gives ammunition to critics, and unfortunately, they're right about some of it.

But the issue isn't the concept of IgG testing. The issue is that we're not doing it well. When labs use validated food antigens, subclass differentiation (especially IgG4 vs IgG1-3), and reproducible ELISA or immunoblot techniques, the data becomes actionable. These are the panels that begin to show patterns consistent with terrain collapse: high-reactivity foods corresponding to neurologic flares, mast cell activation, gastrointestinal distress, or emotional lability. When interpreted properly, they can reveal which food antigens are driving inflammation, not in isolation, but in the larger context of immune overwhelm, adjuvant exposure, or pathogen priming.

Equally problematic is the clinical ignorance surrounding the concept of oral tolerance itself. Few practitioners, conventional or alternative, have been trained to recognize how the breakdown of mucosal immunity and gut filtering leads to systemic reactivity to food. They don't ask whether the patient has had mold exposure, vaccine injury, chronic viruses, or lymphatic stagnation. They don't see how IgG responses reflect not just diet but the terrain's overall ability to regulate immune memory and resolve exposures. Without this systems-level view, even the best test can be misused.

And finally, patients are often left to interpret these results on their own, without guidance. This can lead to restrictive diets based on fear, not physiology. People remove 30 or 40 foods at once, starve their microbiome, and enter deeper depletion. The panel becomes a punishment, rather than a tool for relief. But that's not the test's failure, it's a failure of support, education, and interpretation.

IgG testing does not fail us. We fail when we refuse to read it through the lens of terrain biology, when we don't demand better labs, and when we don't teach people how to use the information as part of a regenerative protocol. In reality, when used with precision and clinical understanding, IgG panels can be one of the most powerful tools for navigating immune overload, calming neuroinflammation, and restoring relationship with food, one step at a time.

How and When to Use IgG Testing in Terrain Repair

The true power of IgG food sensitivity testing emerges only when it's used in the right phase of healing. It is not a first step, it is a clarifying tool that becomes most accurate and most helpful once terrain repletion has begun. That means gut motility is moving, bowel regularity is restored, micronutrient levels are being rebuilt, and the immune system has begun to calm its hypervigilance. If IgG testing is done too early, when the gut is still leaking, the lymph is stagnant, and the immune system is firing wildly, it will often show everything as reactive. That's not because the test is flawed, but because the terrain is overwhelmed.

Once basic terrain foundations are in place, IgG testing becomes a powerful lens for identifying where immune friction remains. For some individuals, the results will reveal true oral intolerances, foods that provoke such strong immunological reactions that they generate terrain-wide effects: brain fog, fatigue, histamine spikes, joint pain, or nervous system agitation. These foods, when removed temporarily, can lead to profound reductions in inflammation and often rapid improvements in mood, focus, energy, and digestion. This isn't guesswork, it's precision removal of a friction point the immune system is struggling to tolerate.

But IgG testing also serves a second, equally important purpose: it helps identify which foods may be carrying hidden burdens, not because of the food itself, but because of what's riding on it. For example, foods like conventional wheat, soy, oats, peanuts, coffee, strawberries, and corn are often loaded with glyphosate or pesticide residues, which can damage tight junctions in the gut, alter the microbiome, and lead to the loss of oral tolerance. When the immune system reacts to these foods, it may be reacting as much to the chemical signature as the food protein.

The same applies to mold-prone foods, such as nuts, grains, dried fruits, and certain spices. For individuals who have lived in water-damaged buildings, been colonized by mold, or are dealing with chronic inflammatory response syndrome (CIRS), these foods can carry enough mycotoxin residue to keep the terrain in a heightened inflammatory state. Even low-level, ongoing exposure can provoke reactivity, especially if the immune system has already been sensitized.

And in some cases, foods may provoke an IgG reaction because of prior immune priming via adjuvants. For instance, someone who has received a vaccine containing egg protein, yeast extract, or polysorbate-80 may later develop an immune recognition pattern for those foods, not because they're inherently intolerant, but because the immune system has been trained to watch for that antigen. This is particularly relevant in people with autoimmune disorders, PANS/PANDAS history, or post-vaccine terrain destabilization.

For individuals with neuroinflammatory terrain, such as ALS, multiple sclerosis, Parkinson's disease, or post-viral syndromes, IgG reactivity to common foods can reveal an immune system under excessive load. This is equally true for those with mast cell overactivation, histamine intolerance, or autoimmune-driven gut collapse. In all of these cases, the goal is not permanent restriction, but temporary relief: a way to lower the immune static so the body can begin to rebuild tolerance, repair the gut lining, and regain metabolic efficiency.

When IgG panels are used at the right time, and interpreted through a terrain-aware lens, they stop being confusing food lists and become maps of immune distress. They show us where to lighten the load, where to pause exposure, and where the body is asking for relief. They give us clues about the broader environmental burden (chemical, microbial, or immune) that food is simply revealing, not causing.

This makes IgG testing not just useful, but essential in advanced terrain repair protocols. Not as a first step, and never in isolation, but as a tool for fine-tuning the path back to immune tolerance, metabolic flow, and nervous system safety.

How to Interpret IgG Panels Accurately

Reading an IgG food sensitivity panel is not about creating a list of "bad foods", it's about learning to read immune patterns with precision. When viewed through the lens of terrain biology, the results become a kind of immune topography map, showing where the body is being overwhelmed, where tolerance is broken, and where filtration systems are failing to protect the inner environment.

One of the most important rules in interpreting IgG panels is this: the most extreme reactivities matter the most.Foods that show up with very high reactivity, markedly higher than others on the panel, often represent true oral intolerances. These are the foods that, for whatever reason (injection-based priming, adjuvant exposure, pathogen mimicry, or genetic susceptibility), have become immunologically charged in a way that triggers broad systemic symptoms. Removing these high-reactive foods can lead to striking changes: improved cognition, less joint pain, better bowel function, clearer skin, or less anxiety. These results are not placebo, they're the terrain relaxing as a major immune burden is lifted.

On the other hand, when you see clusters of moderate-level reactions, especially across a wide range of foods, grains, fruits, proteins, or herbs, it's usually not because all of these foods are problematic. It's because the gut barrier is leaky, and immune cells are tagging everything they see. In this case, the pattern tells us less about the foods themselves and more about the integrity of the filtration system. These foods may not need to be removed individually. Instead, they point to the need for gut sealing, nervous system calming, and microbiome rebalancing. Often, once the permeability is resolved, these moderate reactivities disappear on follow-up testing.

Minor reactions, especially in highly consumed foods, can reflect immune tagging due to frequency, not intolerance. The immune system sees what it sees often, and if you eat a food every day, it may simply be showing up on the radar. This doesn't mean the food is causing problems. But it may be worth rotating out of the diet temporarily, especially if symptoms seem to fluctuate with it. This is where tracking becomes key.

To interpret any IgG panel accurately, context is everything. Always correlate test results with:

Symptom timing (Do symptoms worsen after eating? How quickly?)

Digestive patterns (Bloating, gas, stools, discomfort)

Cognitive or emotional changes (Brain fog, anxiety, irritability)

Current state of gut integrity (Are you still sealing the gut? Still addressing microbial overgrowth or mold?)

Food journaling data, especially if paired with meal timing, mood, and bowel movements

One of the most powerful insights of terrain-informed IgG interpretation is this: when the primary immune irritants are removed, even temporarily, minor and moderate reactivities often resolve themselves. This doesn't mean the original test was flawed. It means that healing lowers the volume of immune reactivity. Tolerance is not static, it can be rebuilt. IgG patterns that looked dramatic in an inflamed state may calm down completely as the terrain resets.

This is why IgG testing is not a one-time verdict. It's a snapshot of immune confusion, one that can evolve over time. Used wisely, it becomes not a restrictive tool, but a liberating one: a map for reducing the immune burden now, and a guide for restoring food resilience over time.

Why Not All Direct-to-Consumer Tests Are Valid

In recent years, the rise of at-home health testing has given many people access to tools that were once locked behind institutional gatekeeping. While this democratization of data has been a lifeline for some, not all tests are created equal, especially when it comes to IgG food sensitivity panels.

Many of the direct-to-consumer (DTC) IgG kits available online or in stores use generic immunoassays that were not developed with clinical-grade rigor. These panels often lack validated food antigens, quality control in sample handling, or even clear reporting standards. Worse, most offer no breakdown by IgG subclass, meaning they don't distinguish between an inflammatory response (IgG1/IgG3) and a tolerance-associated tagging (IgG4). This dramatically limits interpretability. The result? Panels that look scientific but deliver false positives, false negatives, and confusing scattershot results that lead to fear-based restriction or wasted effort.

Without proper context, and without meaningful data quality, these over-the-counter tests can do more harm than good. They may mislead a patient into believing they're intolerant to dozens of foods, when in reality their gut barrier simply needs repair. Or they may miss significant immune burden altogether by failing to detect subclass-specific inflammation.

By contrast, physician-ordered panels through vetted terrain labs like Mosaic Diagnostics, US Biotek, Vibrant Wellness, or ImuPro are built to support serious clinical interpretation. These tests typically use ELISA or immunoblotting methods, validated antigen libraries, and consistent reporting scales. Some even offer IgG subclass breakdowns, allowing the practitioner to distinguish between true oral intolerance and generalized immune surveillance. When used properly, these panels:

Ensure a higher level of test fidelity and reproducibility

Allow integration with other markers of immune and gut function (e.g., zonulin, histamine, calprotectin, eosinophils, cytokine profiles)

Provide documentation that can be shared with practitioners across disciplines (NDs, nutritionists, MDs, health coaches), enabling a unified care plan

However, the unfortunate truth is that many physicians still dismiss IgG testing entirely, often due to outdated assumptions, poor training, or institutional bias. This creates a bind for patients who are aware something is wrong but are denied access to meaningful diagnostics.

That's why patient-directed ordering remains essential, not as a workaround, but as a tool for self-stewarded healing. If your doctor refuses to explore immune reactivity or belittles the idea of food-driven inflammation, you have the right to pursue testing independently. Platforms like Rupa Health, Direct Labs, and some functional nutrition practices allow you to order physician-grade IgG panels without a gatekeeping MD. This can be the difference between staying stuck and making a breakthrough.

The goal is not to bypass clinical wisdom, but to align with practitioners who understand terrain and who are willing to interpret IgG results not as a list of enemies, but as an evolving map of immune traffic, friction, and overload. Whether accessed through a supportive physician or through a trusted direct platform, the quality of the test still matters, and your interpretation deserves the same standard of care.

Integrating IgG Testing into the Healing Process

When used correctly, IgG food sensitivity testing is not a dietary sentence, it's a strategic snapshot of immune activity, meant to guide the terrain back toward balance. In terrain medicine, the goal is never to eliminate foods forever. It is to understand why the immune system has flagged them in the first place, and how to create conditions that allow tolerance to return.

That means IgG results should guide, not dictate, your next steps. The panel is not a list of forbidden foods. It's a map of immune friction points that, if removed temporarily, may create enough calm in the system to allow deeper repair to take place.

The first step is to identify high-reactivity foods, especially those with extreme IgG elevations that correlate with symptoms like bloating, fatigue, brain fog, or inflammatory pain. These are the foods most likely to reflect true oral intolerance or immune system priming. Eliminating them for a defined period, typically 30 to 90 days, can reduce systemic burden and free up energy for healing. But that elimination is only meaningful if it is paired with deeper terrain repair.

This includes:

Sealing the gut lining with amino acids, fatty acids, mucilaginous herbs, and microbiome-friendly fibers

Calming the immune system through vagal toning, nervous system safety work, and mast cell stabilization

Supporting mitochondrial repair, especially in neurologic terrain, where chronic inflammation has drained the body's energy reserves

Without this terrain-focused support, food elimination becomes a loop of deprivation, not liberation. But when layered into a thoughtful, systems-level protocol, temporary removal of IgG-reactive foods can be transformative. It allows inflammation to settle, absorption to improve, and the immune system to begin the slow process of rebuilding tolerance.

The real measure of success is not how many foods you eliminate, but how many you are eventually able to bring back in without symptoms. And that requires a structured process, not just elimination, but strategic reintroduction once the terrain is stable. Reintroduction helps rebuild immune flexibility, retrain digestive enzymes, and restore psychological ease around food.

This is where IgG testing and terrain medicine converge. The test becomes a starting map, not a final rulebook. It helps you prioritize which foods to pause, and when to focus your energy on repair. It offers an immune-informed, data-backed foundation for what has always been the gold standard in terrain-based nutrition: the elimination and reintroduction protocol, customized to your immune landscape, your symptoms, and your body's timing.

Used in this way, IgG testing becomes an ally, not to restrict your life, but to restore your capacity to live fully, eat joyfully, and heal deeply.

Top Food Allergens and Sensitivities Impacting Gut Health

For people with ALS and similar terrain breakdown patterns, gut inflammation is often a silent but powerful driver of symptoms. One of the most overlooked sources of that inflammation is food, not necessarily from what's missing in the diet, but from what's constantly provoking the immune system.

Food sensitivities and allergies can weaken the intestinal barrier, trigger systemic inflammation, and disrupt the very systems you're trying to heal. Even if you've eaten certain foods your whole life without a noticeable reaction, your terrain may no longer tolerate them. Over time, stress, toxic exposures, or microbial imbalances can cause the immune system to misidentify once-safe foods as threats.

Among the most common culprits are:

Gluten
Gluten, the protein found in wheat, barley, and rye, contains a component called gliadin. For many individuals, especially those with autoimmune tendencies or existing gut issues, gliadin triggers the release of a molecule called zonulin. Zonulin increases intestinal permeability, literally opening up the tight junctions of the gut lining and allowing particles to "leak" into circulation. This can amplify immune reactivity and inflammation system-wide. Gluten hides in many processed foods, sauces, and condiments, even where you wouldn't expect it.

Casein
Casein is the main protein in dairy, and it's a different issue than lactose intolerance. While lactose causes digestive discomfort due to enzyme deficiency, casein can provoke immune responses that lead to inflammation, congestion, and even neurological symptoms in sensitive individuals. For some people, casein cross-reacts with gluten, meaning the immune system confuses one for the other, keeping inflammation alive even if you've already removed gluten. Casein is found in milk, cheese, yogurt, and dairy-based products.

Eggs
Eggs, especially the whites, contain proteins like albumin that are common allergens. In sensitive individuals, these proteins can irritate the gut lining and trigger immune responses. Eggs are also

used widely in processed foods, baked goods, and dressings, making them difficult to track unless carefully avoided.

Yeast

Yeast sensitivity is often overlooked, but it can contribute to gas, bloating, brain fog, skin issues, and more. For those with fungal overgrowth, prior mold exposure, or autoimmune activation, yeast-containing foods may act as fuel for dysbiosis. Yeast is found in breads, pastries, beer, wine, and many fermented products.

Soy

Soy contains both allergenic proteins and phytoestrogens that can disrupt hormonal and immune balance in sensitive individuals. It is also one of the most processed and genetically modified crops, often appearing in packaged foods, meat substitutes, and condiments under names like "soy protein isolate" or "vegetable oil."

Corn

Like soy, corn is ubiquitous in the food supply and often genetically modified. For some people, it can act as a low-grade irritant that contributes to gut inflammation, particularly when consumed in the form of corn syrup, processed cereals, snack foods, or industrial oils.

Peanuts and Tree Nuts

While these are well-known allergens, even minor sensitivities can create systemic stress over time. Inflammation triggered by these proteins may not always show up as anaphylaxis, but can still erode gut health in subtle ways.

Shellfish and Fish

Shellfish allergies are among the most common, and their proteins are highly reactive. Even trace amounts can be enough to provoke a response in sensitive individuals. Cross-contamination is a major issue in restaurants and packaged foods.

Sesame
Sesame is now recognized as a major allergen due to its increasing role in allergic reactions. Found in oils, baked goods, sauces, and toppings, it can be difficult to detect without careful label reading.

Removing these common triggers, even temporarily, can dramatically reduce gut inflammation and allow the intestinal lining to begin sealing. While not everyone will be sensitive to all of these foods, doing a focused elimination, combined with terrain repair, can help identify which ones are quietly contributing to collapse.

Additional Gut Irritants to Consider

While food allergens and sensitivities get most of the attention, they're not the only players disrupting gut health. In a terrain that's already inflamed, depleted, or leaky, even subtle irritants can add up, blocking progress and keeping the gut-brain-immune axis in a reactive state. For those healing from ALS or related neurodegenerative conditions, it's especially important to reduce all sources of digestive and immune stress.

Several common but often overlooked irritants include:

Artificial Additives and Preservatives
Artificial colors, sweeteners, emulsifiers, and preservatives are found in many packaged and processed foods, even in items marketed as "natural" or "healthy." These compounds may alter the gut microbiota, weaken the intestinal barrier, and trigger low-grade immune activation. For individuals with already-compromised digestion, these ingredients can silently disrupt the healing process by promoting dysbiosis or fueling systemic inflammation. Removing them is a simple but powerful step toward a calmer terrain.

Alcohol and Caffeine

While socially normalized, both alcohol and caffeine place strain on the gut, and on the nervous system. Alcohol is directly irritating to the gut lining and impairs liver function, which is already under pressure in ALS terrain. Caffeine, while offering short-term alertness, can disrupt digestion, raise cortisol, deplete minerals, and contribute to a stress-based metabolic state. Reducing or eliminating these substances helps the terrain focus on repair rather than reaction.

Nightshade Vegetables (e.g., Tomatoes, Peppers, Eggplants, Potatoes)

Nightshades contain a group of compounds called alkaloids, like solanine and capsaicin, that can be inflammatory or irritating for some individuals, particularly those with autoimmune tendencies or sensitive guts. While not inherently harmful for everyone, those with leaky gut, joint pain, or neurological symptoms may find symptom relief by removing nightshades for a time and reintroducing them cautiously later.

These irritants aren't necessarily problematic in a robust, resilient terrain, but in the context of ALS and systemic breakdown, they can quietly keep the gut inflamed. Removing them creates space for deeper healing, better absorption, and a calmer immune system.

Strategies for Eliminating Trigger Foods

Eliminating trigger foods isn't about jumping onto the latest diet trend or cutting out foods at random. It's a clinical strategy to calm the immune system, reduce inflammation, and allow the gut lining to begin healing. The process, often called an "elimination and reintroduction protocol," is one of the most useful terrain tools you can apply, because it puts the power of discovery in your hands.

Here's how to do it safely and effectively:

Step 1: The Elimination Phase
Start by removing the most common irritants and allergens from your diet, foods like gluten, casein (dairy), eggs, soy, corn, peanuts, yeast, and artificial additives. For individuals with more severe inflammation or immune reactivity, you may also remove nightshades, caffeine, alcohol, and processed sugars. This phase lasts about 3 to 4 weeks.

This time frame is long enough for immune responses to begin quieting and for inflammation to settle. Don't expect immediate results, sometimes symptoms worsen before they improve as the body recalibrates. The goal isn't perfection, but consistency. Even a 90% reduction can offer major insight and relief.

Step 2: Observation
As you move through the elimination phase, begin paying closer attention to how your body responds. Improvements may show up in surprising ways: less bloating, fewer headaches, deeper sleep, calmer mood, better skin, more stable energy. These are signs that the immune system is settling and the gut lining is no longer under constant assault.

You're not just "on a diet." You're running a terrain experiment, one that tells you which foods are keeping your nervous system on high alert.

Step 3: The Reintroduction Phase
After the elimination period, start adding foods back in, one at a time, every 3 to 5 days. This slow reintroduction gives the body time to mount any reactions, which may be delayed (appearing as symptoms the next day, not always immediately).

When reintroducing, choose the food in its most basic, whole form, like a plain boiled egg, a small amount of organic yogurt, or one slice of gluten-containing bread. Avoid mixing ingredients, so you can clearly observe what's causing a reaction.

Step 4: Documentation
Keeping a food and symptom journal is essential. Write down what you eat and how you feel for 24 to 72 hours afterward. Note changes in digestion, sleep, mood, focus, skin, and joint pain. Even subtle reactions, like a slight increase in anxiety or brain fog, can be clues to immune irritation.

This isn't about following strict rules forever. It's about gathering information your body has been trying to give you for years. Once you identify which foods are problematic, you can make empowered choices, whether that means long-term removal, rotation, or finding better-tolerated alternatives.

Ultimately, this process teaches you how to listen to your terrain and feed it with care.

Supportive Foods for Gut Healing

When the goal is to calm the gut and restore the intestinal lining, food becomes more than nourishment, it becomes medicine. But in a fragile terrain, not all "healthy" foods are helpful. Raw salads, cold smoothies, or rough fibrous snacks may overwhelm an already inflamed or leaky digestive system.

Instead, the focus should be on warm, gentle, mucosal-supportive foods, those that soothe rather than stimulate, nourish rather than challenge. These foods help rebuild the intestinal lining, support the microbiome, and allow nutrients to be better absorbed. They also reduce the likelihood of triggering immune reactions during this sensitive phase.

Among the most healing foods are:

Bone Broth

Properly prepared bone broth is one of the most foundational gut-repair foods. When made from organic, pasture-raised bones simmered over many hours, it becomes rich in gelatin, collagen, and amino acids like glutamine and glycine. These compounds directly support the integrity of the gut lining, reduce inflammation, and provide fuel for the cells that repair intestinal tissue. Bone broth is also hydrating and easy to digest, making it ideal for those with poor appetite or absorption issues.

Fermented Foods (if tolerated)
Fermented foods like sauerkraut, kimchi, coconut yogurt, and beet kvass can offer natural sources of beneficial bacteria that help rebalance the gut microbiome. But timing matters. For those with significant histamine issues, small intestinal bacterial overgrowth (SIBO), or mold sensitivity, fermented foods may need to be introduced later, once gut calm has been achieved. When tolerated, they act as gentle microbiome fertilizers, encouraging diversity and immune balance.

Cooked Vegetables
Lightly steamed, roasted, or simmered vegetables provide essential vitamins, minerals, and prebiotic fibers without overstimulating digestion. Cooking breaks down plant fibers, making nutrients easier to absorb and reducing the risk of bloating or irritation. Root vegetables like carrots, beets, and sweet potatoes are especially grounding, while squashes, zucchini, and greens provide a broad spectrum of healing phytonutrients.

Omega-3 Rich Foods
Omega-3 fatty acids help modulate inflammation and support the health of cell membranes, including the cells lining the gut. While cold-water fish like wild salmon or sardines are excellent sources, plant-based omega-3s like chia seeds, flaxseeds, and walnuts can also be helpful. These foods provide alpha-linolenic acid (ALA),

which the body can convert, albeit inefficiently, into EPA and DHA, the more active anti-inflammatory forms.

During this phase, think comfort, warmth, and nourishment. Each meal should feel like it's saying to your body, "You're safe now. You can begin to heal."

Supplementation (As Needed)

Gut Lining Repair

L-Glutamine

> Primary fuel source for intestinal epithelial cells; supports regeneration of a damaged gut lining and reduces permeability ("leaky gut").

> Recommended: Pure Encapsulations L-Glutamine Powder (start with small doses and monitor sensitivity).

Zinc Carnosine

> Synergistic compound that adheres to ulcerated or inflamed gut tissue, promoting healing and reducing mucosal inflammation.

> Recommended: Integrative Therapeutics Zinc-Carnosine.

Digestive Enhancement

Digestive Enzymes

> Aid the breakdown of proteins, fats, and carbohydrates; essential for those with poor digestion, low stomach acid, or bloating after meals.

> Recommended: Pure Encapsulations Digestive Enzymes Ultra or Douglas Labs Enzyme Complex.

Betaine HCl (if tolerated)

Restores stomach acid levels in hypochlorhydria, improving protein digestion and sterilizing incoming pathogens.

Caution: Only use if tested for low stomach acid and not with ulcers or NSAID use.

Recommended: Pure Encapsulations Betaine HCl with Pepsin.

Microbiome Restoration

Targeted Probiotics

Reintroduce beneficial bacteria to rebalance gut flora, reduce inflammation, and outcompete pathogens.

Recommended: Pure Encapsulations Probiotic G.I. or Integrative Therapeutics Pro-Flora Intensive.

Prebiotics (if tolerated)

Feed commensal bacteria and support short-chain fatty acid production.

Use with caution in SIBO or active dysbiosis.

Recommended: Pure Encapsulations Prebiotic Fiber (Partially Hydrolyzed Guar Gum).

Biofilm and Histamine Support

Serrapeptase or NAC

Break down biofilms that protect pathogens in the gut lining and reduce inflammatory debris.

Recommended: Integrative Therapeutics NAC or Douglas Labs Serrapeptase.

DAO or Low-Histamine Support

For those reacting to fermented foods or experiencing

histamine flares, temporary support may help.

Recommended: Pure Encapsulations HistDAO.

Soothing and Anti-inflammatory Compounds

Aloe Vera (inner leaf only)

Calms inflammation and soothes the gut lining.

Recommended: Pure Encapsulations Aloe 200x.

Deglycyrrhizinated Licorice (DGL)

Supports mucosal barrier repair and lowers inflammatory cytokines.

Recommended: Integrative Therapeutics DGL Ultra.

Emotional and Psychological Considerations

Changing your diet, especially when facing a serious illness like ALS, is never just a physical process. It's deeply emotional. Food is far more than fuel. It's culture, comfort, memory, and meaning. Removing long-loved foods can trigger grief, resistance, or even identity crises. It's important to honor this.

For many, the foods that now contribute to inflammation or gut distress are the same ones that brought joy or comfort in times of stress. Bread at family dinners. Creamy sauces tied to childhood. Celebratory desserts. When these foods become harmful, there's a real sense of loss, one that deserves attention, not dismissal.

That's why emotional support is essential when making major dietary changes. This isn't about willpower or perfection. It's about re-patterning deeply ingrained habits in a way that feels respectful and sustainable. For some, that may mean working with a trauma-informed nutritionist or therapist who understands both the biology and psychology of change. For others, simply talking with a loved one or joining a support group can make a profound difference.

Mindfulness practices, like deep breathing before meals, journaling food and mood patterns, or simply noticing emotions that arise when certain foods are removed, can also be powerful tools. These practices help shift the nervous system out of fight-or-flight and into rest-and-digest, where healing actually happens.

The goal isn't restriction. It's restoration. And restoration doesn't require you to be perfect, it asks that you be honest, supported, and compassionate with yourself as you relearn how to nourish your body from a new place of awareness. Over time, this process becomes empowering. Your food choices start to feel less like deprivation and more like devotion to your healing.

Chapter 8: Open the Drainage Pathways

Why Drainage Must Precede Detox

In the world of natural medicine, there's a common mistake that even experienced practitioners make: jumping straight into detoxification. It sounds intuitive, if someone is sick, overloaded, or neurologically deteriorating, the goal should be to remove what's harming them, right?

But in ALS and other fragile terrain conditions, this can backfire in dangerous ways.

Here's the critical distinction: detox is not the same as drainage.

Detox is the process of mobilizing toxins, pulling them out of storage in the liver, fat, bones, or nervous system. That might happen through chelation, fasting, aggressive supplements, or other "detox" protocols. And while mobilizing may seem productive, it's actually hazardous if the body's drainage systems aren't fully open.

Drainage is the excretion of those mobilized toxins. It's the actual removal, the way toxins leave the body through the bowels, kidneys, sweat, lymph, and breath. Without that exit, mobilized toxins have nowhere to go. They simply recirculate.

In ALS terrain, where mitochondria are already overworked and nerves are hypersensitive, this can lead to serious consequences:

A spike in neuroinflammation

Intensified fatigue or weakness

Flare-ups in tremors, spasms, or emotional dysregulation

Even accelerated degeneration in some cases

That's why every effective terrain protocol begins with a simple but non-negotiable rule: "No drainage, no removal. No removal, no relief."

Opening the drainage pathways is not optional, it's foundational. You must clear the exits before you start stirring up stored toxins. You must help the body sweat, urinate, defecate, and release through lymph and skin, before you support the liver in detoxification, before you use binders, and certainly before you chelate.

Think of it like unclogging a sink. If the pipes are blocked, dumping more water in doesn't help, it floods the system. The same is true with terrain healing. You have to open the pipes first.

In the next sections, we'll walk through the major drainage organs, how to support them gently, and what signs show that your exits are ready for deeper detox work.

Overview of the Five Drainage Pathways

Drainage isn't just one system. It's a symphony of excretory processes working together to keep the body clean, clear, and functioning. When we talk about opening drainage pathways, we're talking about supporting multiple channels, each with its own rhythm, responsibilities, and vulnerabilities. If any one of these systems is blocked, burdened, or neglected, the whole detox process can stall or turn toxic.

Let's walk through each of the five major drainage pathways, what they do, and what happens when they're not flowing well.

Bile and Bowels: The Primary Exit Route

The liver plays a central role in detoxification, filtering the blood, neutralizing toxins, and packaging them for removal. Once the liver processes a toxin, it binds it to bile acids and sends it down to the digestive tract, where it should exit the body via stool. But if bile isn't flowing properly, or if bowel movements are slow or irregular, those toxins linger. Worse, they can be reabsorbed through the gut wall and sent back into circulation, triggering more inflammation and neurological stress.

Clues that bile or bowel function is compromised include:

Constipation, or the sensation of incomplete elimination

Pale or clay-colored stools (a sign of poor bile flow)

Bloating or discomfort after eating fatty foods

Coated tongue or persistent bad breath, which can indicate sluggish digestion and liver congestion

Before any formal detox can begin, this channel must be moving freely. Daily, complete bowel movements are a foundational prerequisite for safe healing.

Kidneys: The Fluid Filtration System

The kidneys filter over 50 gallons of blood per day, removing water-soluble waste and toxins through urine. But this process depends on hydration, mineral balance, and overall kidney integrity. When the body is dehydrated, under-mineralized, or inflamed, kidney function slows, and the ability to clear waste products suffers.

Early signs of kidney strain may include:

Dark or low-volume urine despite drinking fluids

Swelling in the hands, feet, or under the eyes

Deep fatigue, especially in the morning or after activity

Rehydration with mineral-rich water, alongside kidney-supportive herbs like nettle or dandelion leaf, can gently restore this pathway.

Lymphatic System: The Waste Highway of the Immune System

The lymphatic system is the body's sewage and surveillance network. It collects cellular debris, toxins, pathogens, and immune waste from every tissue, moving it through lymph nodes for processing before final elimination. Unlike the circulatory system, lymph has no pump. It relies on movement, especially muscle contraction, deep breathing, and fascia glide, to flow.

When the lymph stagnates, waste accumulates. Immune cells become overactivated, and inflammation can surge.

Common signs of lymphatic stagnation include:

Swollen or tender lymph nodes (in the neck, armpits, or groin)

Puffy face, hands, or ankles

Brain fog or sluggish thinking

Sensitivity to temperature or heat intolerance

Gentle movement, breathwork, dry brushing, and lymphatic herbs can encourage flow, but only after the bowels and kidneys are primed to carry waste out.

Fascia: The Structural and Signaling Matrix

Fascia is the body's connective web, wrapping muscles, nerves, and organs in a continuous sheet of communication. Healthy fascia is pliable, hydrated, and responsive. But when inflamed, dehydrated, or traumatized (physically or emotionally), fascia stiffens. This rigidity blocks both lymphatic flow and nerve conduction, cutting off vital terrain communication and preventing proper drainage.

When fascia is "frozen," people often report:

Waking up stiff or taking hours to feel "unlocked"

Pain that seems to migrate unpredictably

Emotional numbness or feeling physically disconnected

Relief from bodywork, craniosacral therapy, or light stretching, indicating that fascia, not just muscle, is involved

Hydration, mineral repletion, fascia-focused bodywork, and consistent movement routines help melt this frozen web and re-enable flow.

Skin: The Emergency Drain

The skin is often considered a backup channel, but in reality, it's a vital part of the body's excretion system. When primary detox organs (like the liver and kidneys) are overwhelmed, the body pushes toxins out through the skin in the form of sweat or eruptions. While this may seem like a superficial issue, chronic skin problems often signal deeper metabolic congestion.

Skin-based symptoms of poor drainage include:

Rashes, acne, or eczema that worsen with stress or detox attempts

Excessive sweating (especially night sweats) or the inability to sweat

Persistent body odor or unusual heat intolerance

Opening the skin for drainage can involve sauna therapy, Epsom salt baths, castor oil packs, or simply increasing healthy sweat through movement. But again, these strategies must wait until the core exits, bowels, kidneys, and lymph, are moving smoothly.

Each of these pathways is interconnected. Think of them like drainage ditches on a farm: if one backs up, the others get overwhelmed. That's why in terrain-based healing, you never detox in isolation. You open all the exits, gently and in the right order, so the body can do what it's designed to do, release, repair, and rebalance.

How to Begin Opening Drainage

Once you understand the importance of drainage, and the five pathways involved, the next question becomes: where do you start? The answer is simple but often overlooked: start slow.

In terrain-based medicine, we don't push detox first. We prepare the exits. This is like priming the pumps before draining a flooded system. You wouldn't blast open the reservoir gates before making sure the downstream channels are clear. Similarly, you don't begin mobilizing toxins until your body has demonstrated it can excrete them safely and consistently.

Below are key ways to begin gently opening drainage without triggering flares or overwhelming the terrain.

Hydration: The First Drainage Signal

Water is the most overlooked detox tool, and the most essential. Without adequate hydration, none of the drainage pathways function efficiently. Lymph thickens, bile stagnates, kidneys strain, and fascia dries out. But not all hydration is created equal.

Plain water alone may not be enough in a depleted system. Mineral-rich hydration helps restore electrolyte balance and charge the water in a way that makes it usable by cells. Start your day and continue throughout with:

A pinch of sea salt or trace mineral drops in filtered water

Herbal infusions like nettle, dandelion leaf, and hibiscus, which add minerals and gently support liver and kidney function

Fresh lemon or aloe vera juice to soothe the gut and stimulate mild bile release

This is foundational. All drainage work begins with cellular hydration.

Binders: Internal Clean-Up Crew

Once bile flow and bowel regularity are established, binders become essential allies in terrain repair. They intercept toxins in the gut, especially those dumped via bile, preventing reabsorption and systemic flare-ups. Below is a list to customize based on constitution, toxin burden, and tolerance.

Psyllium Husk (Soluble Fiber Binder)

> Best for: Sweeping the colon, regulating bowel movements, supporting microbiome terrain.

> Not ideal for: Severe motility issues or low fluid intake.

> Additional role: Prebiotic effect; helps escort toxins already mobilized by other binders. Can be layered with chlorella or clay.

Activated Charcoal

> Best for: Acute reactions, gas, die-off, alcohol or food poisoning.

> Not ideal for: Long-term use without breaks; can constipate and deplete nutrients.

> Tip: Best pulsed when symptoms spike or after known exposures.

Citrus Pectin (Modified Citrus Pectin)

> Best for: Sensitive individuals, gentle daily binding, heavy metals (especially lead and arsenic).

> Not ideal for: Rapid or intense detox demands.

> Bonus: Also lowers galectin-3, linked to fibrosis and neuroinflammation.

Chlorella (Broken Cell Wall)

Best for: Mercury, mold toxins, light daily detox with added mitochondrial support.

Not ideal for: Mold-sensitive, high histamine, or MCAS-prone individuals.

Extra support: High in chlorophyll, magnesium, and RNA building blocks.

Bentonite Clay

Best for: Strong ionic binding, parasites, pesticides, radioactive elements.

Not ideal for: Those with constipation or poor hydration.

Tip: Best cycled with rest periods. Always follow with water.

Zeolite (Clinoptilolite)

Best for: Mycotoxins, ammonia, mold illness, glyphosate.

Not ideal for: Those with kidney issues if not micronized and well-formulated.

Note: Binds selectively based on molecular size and charge; works best in nano or micronized liquid form.

Fulvic & Humic Acids

Best for: Cellular detox, nutrient transport, viral/toxin modulation.

Not ideal for: Use alongside iron supplements; may chelate and interfere.

Bonus: Support mitochondrial respiration and cell membrane permeability.

Apple Pectin (Non-Modified)

Best for: Mild daily detox, gut soothing, cholesterol management.

Not ideal for: High-potency heavy metal needs.

Supportive role: Natural fiber binder with microbiome-enhancing properties.

Enterosgel (Polymethylsiloxane Polyhydrate)

Best for: Sensitive or reactive individuals (MCAS, IBS, histamine intolerance).

Not ideal for: North American availability (limited access).

Unique action: Binds bacterial endotoxins, histamine, and bile acids without binding minerals.

Bamboo Charcoal

Best for: Similar to activated charcoal, but gentler and potentially more mineral-retentive.

Not ideal for: Long-term use without professional supervision.

Tip: Often better tolerated in sensitive guts.

Silica (e.g., Orthosilicic Acid or Diatomaceous Earth)

Best for: Binding aluminum, strengthening connective tissue, reducing biofilm burden.

Not ideal for: Excessive use without checking kidney function.

Mechanism: Displaces aluminum in tissues and enhances detox from cumulative exposure.

How to Use Binders Safely:

Always begin after daily bowel movements are established.

Take away from food, medications, and essential supplements (1–2 hours apart).

Cycle binders to prevent over-restraining the terrain.

Always hydrate well, many binders are drying or absorb water.

Consider stacking: e.g., chlorella in the morning + psyllium midday + charcoal after reactions.

Bitter Herbs: Fueling Liver and Bile Flow

The liver depends on stimulation to keep bile moving. Bitter herbs act as a wake-up call for sluggish liver function. They're not harsh, they're activating. When taken before meals or in teas throughout the day, bitters help emulsify fats, support digestion, and encourage daily elimination.

Effective bitters include:

Gentian: extremely bitter and best in tincture form

Dandelion root: both bitter and liver-supportive

Burdock: supportive for liver and lymph

Artichoke leaf: enhances bile flow and digestion

You'll know they're working when you salivate more, digestion feels smoother, and bowel movements become more regular. This is the body responding with flow.

Lymphatic Support: Movement Is Medicine

The lymph has no built-in pump, it depends on your breath, movement, and fascia glide to move waste through the system. Fortunately, gentle interventions can go a long way.

Start with:

Dry brushing toward the heart before showers, stimulates superficial lymph flow

Rebounding or walking, even a few minutes a day can re-engage the lymphatic rhythm

Castor oil packs, applied over the liver, abdomen, or neck, these soften fascia and stimulate lymphatic clearance

Fascial release techniques, light foam rolling, craniosacral therapy, or self-massage help soften the connective tissue network and re-open stuck flow

For those seeking a nervous system-lymph combo, pair diaphragmatic breathwork with gentle neck massage to open both vagal and lymphatic flow at once.

Skin and Sweat: The Emergency Exit

When the primary drainage pathways are overloaded, the body sends toxins out through the skin. Instead of suppressing this route (with antiperspirants or harsh creams), you can work with it, gently encouraging sweat-based excretion in ways that don't overwhelm a fragile system.

Options include:

Near-infrared saunas or incandescent heat bulbs, low-EMF, mild heat that activates sweat without cardiovascular strain

Epsom salt baths, 2 cups per tub, soak for 20–30 minutes to encourage detox through skin and support magnesium replenishment

Clay baths or foot soaks, help pull heavy metals and toxins from deeper tissues

Natural sweat activation, wearing extra layers during a walk or stretching in a warm room can gently coax sweating

Always pair these methods with hydration and binders to ensure that what's being released isn't just reabsorbed.

Each of these steps begins a conversation with the terrain. You're not forcing detox, you're clearing the exits, signaling safety, and preparing the system to do what it's biologically designed to do: release what it no longer needs. When done in the right order, drainage isn't just safe, it's transformative.

Cautions for ALS Terrain

In the world of chronic illness, "detox" has become a buzzword, often misunderstood and misapplied. For individuals with ALS, the risks of pushing detoxification too early or too aggressively are especially high.

This is not a terrain that can afford violent interventions.

By the time ALS symptoms emerge, the system is already profoundly fragile: mitochondrial output is diminished, the nervous system is hyperreactive or shut down, and drainage pathways are typically impaired. Introducing binders, saunas, chelators, or even certain herbs without proper foundation can backfire, not because those tools are inherently harmful, but because the terrain isn't ready.

Drainage is not the same as purging. We are not forcing elimination, we are reestablishing natural exits. That means coaxing function back into flow, not squeezing it out.

Before even considering detox strategies, these three fundamentals must be in place and stable:

Regular bowel movements (1–2 per day): This is non-negotiable. If the gut is not moving, toxins released from the liver or lymph will simply get reabsorbed, worsening inflammation and symptom burden.

Warm, mineralized hydration: Hydration must include trace minerals and salts to support cellular transport and detox. Cold water and overhydration without minerals can dilute electrolytes and stress the kidneys.

Gentle lymphatic and fascia movement: Think circulation, not exertion. Light dry brushing, castor oil packs, walking, or cranial release techniques help the fascia "unfreeze" and lymph flow resume, without overwhelming a sensitive system.

Most importantly, listen to the body. If symptoms flare, such as increased muscle fasciculations, fatigue, anxiety, rashes, or digestive disruption, stop. This is a message from the terrain: it's not ready to release. In these moments, always return to the basics:

Prioritize hydration

Reduce or pause binders, bitters, or sweating practices

Reintroduce mineral and mitochondrial support

In terrain medicine, healing happens by capacity, not by force. What you can eliminate safely is only as great as what you've restored. And that restoration takes time, rhythm, and a deep respect for the body's innate pace.

Terrain-Safe Drainage Starter Routine (Example)

For anyone living with ALS terrain or similar chronic conditions, the idea of "drainage" might sound abstract or clinical, but in truth, it's a deeply biological rhythm. Opening the body's drainage pathways isn't about doing everything at once or pursuing extreme interventions. It's about restoring the natural flow of elimination that your body already wants to do, if only it were gently supported.

This simple routine is designed to match the body's natural rhythm across the day. Think of it as a daily conversation with your terrain: waking it up, keeping it supported, and preparing it to release.

In the morning, begin by waking your cells with hydration that actually reaches them. A warm glass of water with a pinch of sea salt and a squeeze of fresh lemon not only stimulates peristalsis, the movement of your intestines, but also primes the liver and kidneys. The lemon offers gentle liver stimulation, while the salt helps drive hydration into the cells instead of simply passing through.

Next, consider applying a castor oil pack to the abdomen or performing a short dry brushing session before your shower. Castor oil has been used for centuries to gently activate lymphatic flow and reduce local inflammation. Dry brushing, especially in the direction of the heart, stimulates surface lymph and fascia, setting the stage for better drainage throughout the day.

At midday, just before lunch, take a small dose of herbal bitters. These taste pungent for a reason: they stimulate your vagus nerve, which helps trigger bile release and supports digestion from top to bottom. This bitter signal is one of the most primal and terrain-supportive tools we have. It tells the liver and gallbladder to get moving, no force, just reminder.

To maintain fluid filtration through the kidneys and liver, sip on a mineral-rich herbal tea throughout the afternoon. Nettle and dandelion leaf are two of the best options. They are gentle diuretics that don't deplete minerals, while also nourishing the blood, lymph, and adrenals. Think of these herbs not as medications, but as ancient allies in reactivating the body's own waste-clearing systems.

In the evening, only if your bowel movements are already regular and well-formed, you can begin introducing a gentle binder. Citrus pectin or chlorella are ideal starting points. These substances act like tiny sponges, grabbing toxins that have entered the digestive tract via bile and escorting them safely out. Timing matters: take your binder away from food, medications, or other supplements, so it doesn't interfere with their absorption.

As you prepare for sleep, support your secondary drainage pathway, the skin. An Epsom salt foot soak (using magnesium sulfate) can draw toxins through the skin while also calming the nervous system and replenishing magnesium. Alternatively, or in addition, use a near-infrared light over your chest and neck to stimulate lymphatic movement and mitochondrial activity in fascia-dense regions.

The goal here is not to detox, it's to prepare the terrain. This routine signals to your body that it is safe, supported, and hydrated. That message is the beginning of real healing.

Chapter 9: Identify and Reduce Toxin Inputs

Why Exposure Reduction Is Non-Negotiable

For many people, the first instinct after receiving an ALS diagnosis, or any serious chronic condition, is to look for ways to "get toxins out." This is understandable. Detox has become a buzzword, and there's no doubt that environmental toxins play a role in neurological decline. But what's often missed is this: removal alone won't work if you're still adding fuel to the fire.

In terrain medicine, reducing toxic input is not a side strategy. It's the foundation. No matter how carefully you support detoxification or how many binders or chelators you take, if new toxins continue entering the system daily, healing can't fully take hold. It's like trying to dry out a flooded basement while the pipe is still leaking.

Toxins, whether they come from moldy buildings, heavy metals in cookware or fillings, pesticides in food, or volatile compounds in cleaning products, don't just accumulate in tissues. They actively disrupt biology as they go. They inflame mitochondria, damage nerve membranes, impair oxygen use, trigger autoimmune responses, and overload drainage pathways. For people with ALS, whose terrain is already fragile and inflamed, even low-level exposures can tip the system toward further dysfunction.

That's why exposure reduction is non-negotiable. It's not about living in fear or becoming obsessive. It's about making smart, terrain-safe choices that reduce the burden on your body, so it can finally shift into healing mode.

Even modest steps, like filtering your drinking water, switching to non-toxic cleaning and personal care products, and addressing obvious sources of mold or chemical exposure in the home, can profoundly reduce inflammation. The terrain begins to calm. The nervous system starts to stabilize. And only then can detox, regeneration, and repair actually begin.

In ALS, the first question is not "how do I detox?" It's "how do I stop the inflow?"

Core Toxin Categories That Disrupt Terrain

One of the most overlooked truths in neurodegenerative conditions like ALS is that many of the symptoms we associate with "disease progression" may, in fact, be the terrain reacting to chronic toxin exposure. These exposures can be subtle and constant, background noise in the body's biology. Over time, they become overwhelming. If the terrain is already inflamed, nutrient-depleted, and struggling to maintain mitochondrial function, even small amounts of exposure can tip the balance toward dysfunction.

To reclaim healing capacity, we must first identify and reduce the most common categories of environmental toxins. Each of these creates unique stress on the terrain, but together, they form a web that suffocates mitochondrial repair, destabilizes nerve signaling, and blocks detox pathways. Here's what to look for:

Mold and Mycotoxins

Toxic mold isn't just an allergy issue, it's a neurological one. The toxins released by certain mold species (mycotoxins) are profoundly disruptive to mitochondrial energy production and immune regulation. Mold doesn't have to be visible or musty-smelling. It thrives in hidden places: behind drywall, in HVAC ducts, under floors, or in old books and upholstery.

People with mold illness often experience symptoms that overlap with ALS terrain collapse: brain fog, chronic fatigue, dizziness, light or sound sensitivity, chemical intolerance, and sinus congestion. The nervous system becomes hyper-reactive. Detox becomes nearly impossible. And mitochondrial function plummets.

Mold exposure must always be ruled out early. In terrain collapse, it's often the invisible insult keeping the body locked in a loop of inflammation and degeneration.

Heavy Metals

Heavy metals like mercury, lead, aluminum, and arsenic do not exit the body easily. They accumulate slowly over time and embed themselves in fatty tissues, bone, and nerves, particularly in individuals with sluggish detox pathways or low glutathione levels.

These metals directly damage mitochondria by disrupting their respiratory chain. They interfere with antioxidant enzymes, weaken detox organs like the liver and kidneys, and mimic essential minerals, causing confusion at the cellular level. Symptoms include muscle weakness, tremors, memory issues, numbness, and chronic fatigue, all of which mirror ALS.

The most common sources are dental fillings (mercury), contaminated fish, lead pipes, aluminum cookware or deodorants, and rice or drinking water tainted with arsenic. Even small, cumulative exposures can poison the terrain. Identifying and reducing exposure is a critical first move before chelation or detox.

Pesticides and Herbicides

Modern agricultural chemicals like glyphosate (the active ingredient in Roundup) and organophosphates are potent disruptors of terrain health. They compromise the gut microbiome, weaken the blood-brain barrier, impair the liver's detox enzymes, and mimic acetylcholine, a neurotransmitter vital for muscle movement and brain function.

These compounds are sprayed not just on produce but on grains, lawns, and even public parks. Glyphosate residues are nearly ubiquitous in the food supply. For ALS patients, repeated exposure is particularly harmful, studies have found a higher incidence of ALS among farmers and those living in rural, chemically treated environments.

Reducing exposure by choosing organic, filtering water, and avoiding lawn chemicals may seem simple, but these actions profoundly reduce the body's inflammatory burden.

Volatile Organic Compounds (VOCs)

Many people don't realize their homes or workplaces may be contributing to toxic overload. VOCs are chemicals that off-gas from products like paints, adhesives, cleaning sprays, air fresheners, candles, new carpets, and even furniture.

These airborne toxins are inhaled and absorbed through the skin and lungs. They inflame the sinuses, burden the liver, and reduce oxygen transport. Over time, they disturb sleep, create "wired and tired" fatigue, and exacerbate neuroinflammation.

The body terrain affected by ALS is often exquisitely sensitive to VOCs, even mild exposure can trigger flares. Scented products labeled "fresh" or "clean" are among the worst offenders. A toxin-aware home must begin with air quality.

Pharmaceuticals

While medications are often necessary in acute settings, many chronically used drugs add significant weight to the toxic load, especially in vulnerable terrain. Common culprits include:

Statins, which deplete CoQ10, harming mitochondrial function.

Proton-pump inhibitors (PPIs), which reduce stomach acid, hindering nutrient absorption and raising infection risk.

NSAIDs, which damage the gut lining and increase systemic inflammation.

Anticholinergics, which impair memory and cognition, compounding neurological decline.

A comprehensive medication review with a knowledgeable practitioner can identify which drugs may be contributing to terrain stress. Reducing or substituting these safely is often a turning point in healing.

EMFs and Electrical Stressors

Though not chemical, electromagnetic fields (EMFs) and wireless radiation exert real biological effects on terrain health. EMFs can open calcium channels in cell membranes, destabilize mitochondrial ATP production, and disrupt the circadian rhythm, especially when exposures are constant and close to the body.

Devices like Wi-Fi routers, Bluetooth speakers, wireless beds, smart meters, and phones kept near the body (especially at night) create a field of energetic interference. In ALS terrain, where the nervous system is already overexcitable and fragile, these stressors can worsen sleep, anxiety, twitching, and inflammation.

Reducing EMF exposure, especially during sleep, is one of the most powerful and underappreciated strategies to reduce terrain agitation and restore deep repair cycles.

Together, these six toxin categories form the modern terrain challenge.
And for anyone seeking true neurological repair, the message is clear: before you detox, first stop the flood.

How to Identify Toxin Sources in Daily Life

Before you can meaningfully reduce your exposure to toxins, you have to know where they're coming from, and often, the biggest culprits are hiding in plain sight. Most people think of toxins as things "out there": industrial sites, car exhaust, or big chemical spills. But in reality, the most impactful exposures usually come from the environments we occupy every day, especially our homes.

Start with your living space. The average person spends more than 90% of their time indoors, and that means your home environment may be silently shaping your terrain for better or worse. If your house has any history of water damage, even a leak that was "fixed" years ago, it may be harboring hidden mold behind walls or under floors. Poor ventilation, especially in modern airtight homes, traps VOCs from cleaning products, furniture, and synthetic building materials. Scented candles, plug-in air fresheners, dryer sheets, and flame-retardant sofas all release chemicals that burden your liver and destabilize your nervous system, even if they smell "clean."

Then turn to your food. Pesticide residues on non-organic produce, glyphosate-laced grains, and heavily processed or plastic-packaged snacks introduce daily toxins to an already burdened gut-liver system. Repeated exposure to artificial additives, preservatives, emulsifiers, and food dyes doesn't just disrupt digestion, they confuse the immune system and create low-grade inflammation that feeds neurodegeneration. Even cookware matters: nonstick pans, plastic containers, and aluminum foil all leach compounds that interfere with hormonal and mitochondrial function.

Check your bathroom and self-care products. Many conventional toiletries are formulated with known endocrine disruptors, synthetic fragrances, petroleum derivatives, and preservatives like parabens or formaldehyde-releasing agents. These may seem trivial, but remember, what goes on your skin goes into your system. Start scanning labels on items like toothpaste, deodorant, shampoo, lotion, sunscreen, and cosmetics. When possible, switch to cleaner brands that disclose full ingredient lists and avoid synthetic scents.

Next, examine your energy environment. At night, your body enters deep restoration mode, but this only happens when the nervous system feels safe. Blue light exposure from LED bulbs, phones, or screens can delay melatonin release, suppressing immune function and disrupting sleep cycles. Wi-Fi routers, smart devices, and chargers kept near the bed emit electromagnetic fields that subtly agitate the brain and vagus nerve, making it harder to enter parasympathetic healing states. Simple shifts like turning off routers at night, using airplane mode, and swapping harsh LEDs for warmer lighting can make a significant difference.

Finally, review your medications. Many people with complex or chronic health issues are on multiple drugs, but few know that common prescriptions can quietly damage the terrain over time. If you're taking acid blockers, blood pressure meds, mood stabilizers, or cholesterol-lowering drugs, it's worth working with a practitioner to assess which ones may be necessary and which might have safer alternatives. The goal isn't to abandon medical treatment, but to identify where medications might be causing more harm than help, especially in a fragile system.

Toxin reduction doesn't happen all at once. But as you begin to audit and adjust the spaces and inputs that surround you, your terrain receives a powerful message: the inflow has stopped. Only then can the body shift from managing constant injury to reclaiming its power to repair.

Simple Terrain-Safe Strategies to Reduce Toxic Inflow

Reducing toxic input isn't about achieving a sterile life, it's about making mindful swaps that protect your terrain while still allowing you to function in the modern world. For people with ALS and similar terrain-collapse conditions, even small, consistent improvements in environmental exposure can translate into big gains in energy, clarity, and stability over time.

Start with your air. We often think of clean air as something outside, but indoor air quality is what matters most, especially since most people spend the majority of their time indoors. Investing in a high-quality HEPA air filter for your bedroom and main living space can drastically cut your exposure to airborne particulates, mold spores, and volatile organic compounds (VOCs). Try to open windows daily when outdoor air is fresh and pollen counts are low. Just as importantly, eliminate sources of indoor air pollution: skip the plug-in air fresheners, scented candles, incense sticks, and any "fragrance" that doesn't come from real, whole plants. These products release chemical compounds that strain your liver, inflame your brain, and often worsen mitochondrial fatigue.

Next, upgrade your water. Tap water may look clean, but it can carry residues of chlorine, fluoride, heavy metals, pharmaceutical run-off, and agricultural pesticides. A high-quality water filtration system, ideally one that filters both drinking and shower water, is one of the most important investments in terrain health. If budget is a concern, start with a countertop gravity filter that removes chlorine, VOCs, and heavy metals. Don't store filtered water in plastic bottles or jugs; use glass or stainless steel to avoid leaching microplastics and endocrine-disrupting chemicals.

Rethink your kitchen setup. Food and how it's prepared can be either nourishing or damaging, depending on the tools and materials used. Focus on sourcing organic produce when possible, especially those on the Environmental Working Group's "Dirty

Dozen" list, foods that tend to carry the highest pesticide loads. Choose wild-caught or low-mercury fish (like sardines or wild salmon) to avoid adding to your body's metal burden. Ditch Teflon and nonstick pans, which release toxic fumes and chemicals when heated, and instead opt for stainless steel, ceramic, or well-seasoned cast iron. Avoid microwaving anything in plastic wrap or containers, which can release harmful plasticizers into your food.

Be just as careful with what you put on your body as what you put in it. Your skin is a major absorption surface, and conventional personal care products are often loaded with ingredients that interfere with hormone balance, immune function, and liver detox. Choose products made with simple, botanical ingredients, fragrance-free or scented only with essential oils. Use natural deodorants that don't contain aluminum. Replace toothpaste with fluoride-free, SLS-free alternatives that support oral health without disrupting the gut-brain axis. If you use makeup or lotions, seek out brands that are transparent about ingredients and free from parabens, phthalates, and petroleum byproducts.

Don't ignore the mold factor. Mold exposure is often invisible, and deeply destabilizing to the nervous system. If you live in a humid area, a dehumidifier can keep your home's moisture level under 50%, which helps prevent mold growth. Pay special attention to places like basements, attics, and under sinks, spaces where water damage can go unnoticed for years. If you smell musty odors, don't dismiss them. Address leaks immediately and clean any visible mold with non-toxic agents like hydrogen peroxide or vinegar (not bleach, which kills only surface spores and can worsen air toxicity).

Finally, reduce EMF exposure, especially during sleep. While electromagnetic fields (EMFs) may not be as visible as mold or metals, they still act as a form of energetic stress on the terrain.

You don't need to live in a cave or abandon technology, but you can be strategic. Turn off Wi-Fi routers at night or use a timer plug to automate it. Use airplane mode on your phone when carrying it in a pocket or sleeping nearby. Avoid sleeping near smart meters or large electronics, and consider switching to wired devices for your computer or audio equipment when possible.

The goal of these changes is not to create a life of limitation, but to create a life where your body no longer has to fight invisible battles every day. By removing what harms and replacing it with what supports, you free up energy for healing, clarity, and resilience. This is what it means to reduce toxic inflow: fewer assaults on your biology, and more room for your terrain to recover.

This Is About Reducing the Load, Not Perfection

If you're feeling overwhelmed by the idea of reducing toxins, you're not alone. In a world where chemicals are in everything from our toothpaste to our throw pillows, it can feel like a losing battle. But here's the good news: healing doesn't require a perfect, pristine, toxin-free life. It simply requires less, less burden, less inflammation, less disruption to your body's ability to self-regulate and repair.

Terrain medicine isn't about fear, it's about capacity. Every small change you make reduces the load your mitochondria, immune system, and nervous system have to manage. Each filtered glass of water, each switch to a cleaner product, each breath of fresher air gives your terrain one more opportunity to shift from survival into healing.

Start with the obvious. What do you breathe in every day? What touches your skin? What do you drink? Focus your efforts first on high-exposure categories like air, water, food, and sleep environments. These are the daily contacts that either nourish or deplete your terrain.

You don't have to get everything right. You don't need to swap every product overnight. And you certainly don't need to live in fear of the occasional exposure. This isn't about rigidity. It's about momentum.

Your body notices the difference. It responds to consistency, not perfection. The terrain remembers every supportive action, and it builds on them. Over time, what once felt like sacrifice starts to feel like self-respect. What felt like a chore becomes a rhythm. And what felt overwhelming becomes empowering.

This chapter, like the terrain itself, isn't about doing it all, it's about doing what you can, with intention, and letting that be enough. Because it is.

Chapter 10: Calm the Overactive Immune System

Why the Immune System Loses Its Rhythm

In the terrain of ALS, the immune system doesn't simply weaken, it loses its rhythm. What begins as a protective response turns into a confused, overreactive cascade. Instead of acting like a well-trained orchestra responding in harmony, the immune system behaves more like an alarm that never turns off, blaring at everything, useful or not.

This state is often misunderstood. ALS isn't a disease of immune suppression in the way that HIV or chemotherapy might be. Instead, many people with ALS are caught in a terrain pattern of immune hyperactivation, a smoldering fire that won't go out. And that fire starts with chronic, unresolved exposures.

Toxins from mold, heavy metals, and pesticides signal the immune system that something is wrong. Hidden infections, like stealth viruses or intracellular bacteria, push it further. Add to that years, sometimes decades, of unprocessed emotional stress or trauma, and the terrain becomes a battlefield. Over time, immune cells become primed, meaning they respond faster and more aggressively to every perceived threat.

This results in chronic, low-grade inflammation, especially in the brain (neuroinflammation), that damages neurons, impairs mitochondrial energy production, and prevents the body from switching into healing mode. The immune system starts attacking not just foreign invaders, but your own tissues, mistaking broken cells and damaged nerves for threats. This is part of why ALS progresses even when a person starts eating better or taking supplements: the underlying immune confusion hasn't been addressed.

Restoring immune rhythm requires more than immune-boosting. It means calming, retraining, and gently rebalancing the system so that it knows when to activate and when to stand down. It means shifting the terrain from "fight" to "flow." Because in ALS, the goal isn't to strengthen an already aggressive immune response, it's to restore intelligence to it.

Core Immune Imbalances in ALS Terrain

The immune system in ALS terrain doesn't just overreact, it becomes skewed in specific, predictable ways. Certain branches of the immune response become louder, more chaotic, and more destructive, while others go silent or ineffective. Three key imbalances often underlie the chronic inflammation and neurodegeneration seen in ALS and similar terrain collapse patterns: mast cell overactivation, microglial priming, and cytokine dysregulation.

Mast Cell Activation: The Fire Starters

Mast cells are among the immune system's first responders. They're designed to react quickly to potential threats, releasing histamine, cytokines, and other inflammatory chemicals that help defend the body and signal danger. But in the fragile terrain of ALS, these cells often become overactive and trigger-happy.

Rather than reacting only to genuine threats like pathogens or injury, overactivated mast cells may fire off in response to everyday stimuli, foods, temperature changes, EMFs, even emotional stress. The result is a body in a constant low-grade state of alarm. This doesn't just cause itching or sneezing, it can destabilize the nervous system, disrupt digestion, and set off chain reactions throughout the terrain.

People with mast cell activation may experience mysterious symptoms: rashes that appear out of nowhere, sudden fatigue after eating, anxiety or insomnia that doesn't match their situation. Often, these signs are dismissed or misattributed, when in reality they're pointing to a deeper immune regulation failure.

Microglial Priming: The Brain's Hypervigilance

Microglia are the immune cells of the brain and spinal cord. Under normal conditions, they help clean up debris, protect neurons, and support repair. But in ALS terrain, microglia often enter a "primed" state, one where they're constantly on edge, ready to fire at the smallest signal.

This priming often begins years before diagnosis, triggered by viral infections, heavy metal exposure, or gut-brain axis disruption. Once primed, microglia don't just overreact, they begin to release toxic compounds that damage mitochondria, disrupt synapses, and even kill neurons. What's worse, they become poor communicators, responding to local signals but ignoring the terrain's bigger needs.

This chronic microglial hyperactivity is a central driver of neuroinflammation. It contributes to brain fog, irritability, emotional reactivity, and eventually, structural nerve damage. And because microglia respond to both immune and emotional signals, trauma and inflammation become biologically indistinguishable, feeding the loop further.

Cytokine Imbalance: The Lost Language of Immunity

Cytokines are the signaling molecules of the immune system, the "words" immune cells use to coordinate their actions. But in ALS terrain, this chemical language becomes distorted and incoherent. Some cytokines (like IL-6 or TNF-alpha) become overexpressed, keeping inflammation high, while others that help resolve or calm the response become underactive.

When cytokines are out of balance, the immune system can't shut down its response properly. This leads to chronic, non-resolving inflammation that affects the gut, brain, joints, fascia, and mood. The result is often misunderstood symptoms: vague pain, a sense of being feverish without fever, or intense emotional states that feel disproportionate or erratic.

What many people don't realize is that cytokine storms don't have to be acute to be damaging. A slow, simmering imbalance is just as dangerous, especially for neurons, which are highly sensitive to chemical shifts in their environment. Rebalancing cytokines isn't just an immune task, it requires a full terrain recalibration: reducing exposures, supporting mitochondria, and restoring nervous system safety.

Together, these three patterns, mast cell activation, microglial priming, and cytokine imbalance, form the inflammatory backbone of ALS terrain. Left unaddressed, they perpetuate the degeneration. But when understood and gently modulated, they offer a path toward immune restoration and neuroprotection.

How to Calm an Overactive Immune System (Without Suppressing It)

When immune cells stay locked in high-alert mode, the body burns itself out. But calming the immune system isn't the same as suppressing it. Suppression, whether through steroids, immunosuppressant drugs, or blanket antihistamines, can silence important defenses and slow recovery. What the terrain truly needs is immune regulation, not blunt-force muting.

True immune calming begins by understanding that the immune system doesn't operate in a vacuum. It is in constant dialogue with the nervous system, the gut, and the environment. If the terrain is inflamed, unsafe, overexposed, or undernourished, the immune system will continue to overreact, no matter how many anti-inflammatory supplements are taken.

Step 1: Restore Nervous System Safety First

The immune system closely tracks the nervous system's perception of safety. If the brainstem detects threat, whether from trauma, noise, isolation, or pain, immune cells will stay on guard, interpreting everything as danger. This is especially true in ALS terrain, where subtle fear signals can perpetuate inflammation even without an active infection.

To downshift immune alertness, the terrain must feel safe at a cellular level. This starts with daily, terrain-safe practices that calm the vagus nerve and regulate the stress response. Gentle breathwork (with slow, extended exhales), grounding techniques like walking barefoot or connecting to tree bark, and early-morning sunlight exposure all signal "safety" to both the nervous and immune systems.

Touch is another underestimated tool. Whether through self-massage, craniosacral work, or light compression, slow and rhythmic contact reorients the brainstem toward safety, decreasing sympathetic overdrive. For some individuals, trauma-informed modalities like DNRS (Dynamic Neural Retraining System), the Gupta Program, or Primal Trust may help unwind deeply embedded threat patterns and allow the immune system to stand down.

Step 2: Introduce Immune-Calming Herbs and Nutrients

Once the body is no longer in a state of constant alarm, specific botanicals and nutrients can help stabilize immune cells without impairing their function. These are not immunosuppressants, they're immunoregulators. They nudge the system back into balance, especially for those with mast cell activation, cytokine excess, or microglial priming.

Quercetin and luteolin, for example, help stabilize mast cells so they're less likely to degranulate inappropriately. Vitamin C has a natural antihistamine effect while also supporting tissue repair. Omega-3 fatty acids reduce the production of inflammatory cytokines that contribute to "cytokine storms," especially in the nervous system.

Magnesium, particularly in glycinate or threonate forms, soothes both muscles and immune tissues. It's a nervous system mineral, but also a key immune modulator. Trace lithium orotate (in microdose amounts) can stabilize microglia and buffer emotional extremes that worsen inflammation. Gentle herbs like chamomile, skullcap, and holy basilprovide both immune-calming and emotional grounding effects without sedating or suppressing.

Step 3: Consider a Low-Histamine Diet If Symptoms Warrant

Not everyone with ALS terrain needs to avoid histamine-rich foods, but if mast cell activation is suspected, temporary dietary adjustments can make a big difference. Histamine overload tends to cause symptoms like facial flushing, itching after meals, headaches, brain fog, or sinus congestion, especially after eating fermented, aged, or leftover foods.

In such cases, reducing high-histamine foods for several weeks may offer relief. This includes skipping aged cheeses, vinegar, cured meats, kombucha, sauerkraut, and leftovers. Instead, focus on fresh-cooked meals made with simple, whole ingredients.

Support for histamine breakdown (via the DAO enzyme) also matters. Nutrients like vitamin B6, copper, and herbal nettles can help the body degrade excess histamine, easing symptoms without relying solely on avoidance.

Step 4: Support the Gut-Immune Axis

Roughly 70% of the immune system resides in the gut lining. This means gut dysfunction equals immune dysfunction. When the lining is inflamed, leaky, or microbiome-depleted, immune cells lose their tolerance and begin attacking perceived invaders, including foods, microbes, and even self-tissue.

Ongoing gut support is essential. That means continuing to nourish the gut lining with glutamine, zinc carnosine, and collagen-rich foods, while also encouraging healthy microbial diversity. Probiotics may be helpful for some, but they must be introduced carefully, especially in individuals with histamine intolerance or SIBO. Sometimes, just adding a spoonful of fermented vegetable juice (like the brine from fresh sauerkraut) is enough to begin reseeding without triggering reactions.

Finally, keep the bowels moving. Regular elimination via bitters, hydration, and binders prevents recirculation of inflammatory compounds that stress both the liver and immune system.

Step 5: Reduce External Immune Triggers

An immune system constantly bombarded by toxins, mold spores, synthetic chemicals, and EMFs has no chance to calm down. This isn't about fear, it's about giving the immune system a break. Every exposure adds to the load. Every removed irritant creates more space for repair.

Clean water, low-toxin air, and EMF mitigation form the foundation. So does consistent sleep hygiene, since immune function and circadian rhythm are tightly interlinked. Even a 10% improvement in exposure reduction can shift the immune tone, especially when combined with nervous system safety and gut healing.

When you calm without suppressing, the immune system doesn't shut down, it reorients. It stops attacking the self. It starts responding to real threats instead of phantoms. And that shift opens the door to true regeneration.

Emotional Safety as Immune Medicine

The immune system is not merely a biological responder to bacteria, viruses, or toxins, it is an exquisitely sensitive barometer of emotional safety. It listens not just to molecules, but to meaning. To the body, a threat is a threat, whether it's mold exposure, a reactivated virus, or unresolved grief. That's why emotional regulation isn't just mental health care, it's immune care.

In ALS terrain, where the body is already under immense strain, even subtle emotional distress can keep the immune system locked in hypervigilance. Chronic fear, helplessness, or anticipatory grief can flood the system with stress signals that upregulate inflammation, disrupt sleep, impair digestion, and trigger immune flares. When the nervous system perceives danger, the immune system acts accordingly, regardless of whether that danger is physical or emotional.

Healing begins when the terrain receives a different message: you are safe now. And that message must come from more than logic, it has to be felt somatically, viscerally, in the tissues. That's why emotional safety must be cultivated, not just understood.

One of the most powerful ways to support immune regulation is to reframe the illness experience. Instead of interpreting symptoms as betrayal, begin to see them as communication. The body is not attacking itself; it is attempting to signal that something is out of alignment. This shift, from fear to curiosity, from war to listening, can soften the immune response by changing the internal narrative from threat to repair.

Slowing down is another form of medicine. In terrain collapse, the body's pace is often drastically reduced, but the mind may still be racing. Learning to match your mental tempo to the physical body's needs is a form of attunement that creates coherence across systems. It's a way of telling the body: "I'm not abandoning you. I'm here. I'm listening."

Human connection is vital here. The immune system responds profoundly to safe, attuned relationships. Whether that's a caregiver, a loved one, a support group, or even a pet, moments of connection send signals of safety through the vagus nerve, lowering inflammation and increasing immune tolerance.

Finally, emotional safety sometimes requires deeper work. Unprocessed grief, trauma, or shock can continue to reverberate in the immune system until gently resolved. This doesn't mean "thinking positively", it means creating space for emotional digestion. Journaling, somatic experiencing, EMDR (Eye Movement Desensitization and Reprocessing), and trauma-informed therapies can all support this process. These approaches don't just help you feel better emotionally, they actively shift immune tone toward repair and tolerance.

When emotional safety is restored, the immune system can finally stop fighting ghosts. It can come out of defense mode. And in that state of peace, healing isn't just possible, it becomes biologically preferable.

Signs Your Immune System Is Rebalancing

When your immune system begins to come out of hypervigilance and back into rhythm, the change is often quiet, but unmistakable. The body doesn't announce healing with fireworks. It whispers it in small, steady shifts that accumulate over time.

These signs may be subtle at first, but they signal a profound reorientation of the terrain, from inflammation to regulation, from alarm to calm.

One of the first indicators is improved tolerance, to food, light, sound, and environmental stimuli. Where once a bite of fermented food, a sunny day, or a loud room might have triggered discomfort, now these exposures may feel less intense, or even neutral. This isn't a coincidence. It's a reflection of the immune system beginning to discern what is truly threatening and what is not. That discernment is a hallmark of healing.

You may also notice a more stable emotional baseline. The constant swings, between anxiety and collapse, irritability and shutdown, start to soften. You might find yourself responding instead of reacting. This doesn't mean life stops being difficult. It means your system is no longer treating everyday stressors as emergencies. That space between stimulus and response begins to widen, giving you room to breathe.

Sleep deepens. For many navigating ALS or terrain collapse, sleep becomes fragmented, shallow, or unrestorative. As the immune system quiets, so does the nervous system, and with it, the ability to enter deeper stages of rest. You may begin waking up with more clarity, less brain fog, and a sense that your body has done meaningful repair overnight. This is a major sign that inflammation is lowering and mitochondrial repair is underway.

Rashes, itching, flushing, and internal heat often resolve next. These are outward signs of inner immune overdrive, particularly tied to histamine and cytokine imbalances. When they recede, it reflects a more stable mast cell response and less systemic inflammation. Your skin, after all, is often your most visible immune organ, it tells the story of what's going on inside.

And perhaps most telling of all, you may start to feel a sense of physiological "quiet." After meals, instead of bloating, flushing, or fatigue, you may feel calm. After rest, instead of waking with tension or stiffness, there's a softness in the body. This inner quiet is not passive, it's a sign that multiple systems (gut, brain, immune, and fascia) are finally moving together in harmony.

These shifts are not flukes. They are biomarkers of progress. You are not just managing symptoms, you are changing the underlying terrain. And in that new landscape, repair is not just more likely, it becomes the path of least resistance.

Chapter 11: Repair the Barriers That Protect You

Why Barrier Repair Is the Final Sealing Phase

Inside your body are protective membranes so thin they're nearly invisible, yet they are among the most vital defenses you have. These internal barriers are not passive walls; they are intelligent boundaries, constantly evaluating what belongs and what doesn't, regulating flow, filtering toxins, and protecting your most delicate systems from overload and confusion.

Three of these barriers matter most when it comes to ALS and terrain collapse: the gut lining, the blood-brain barrier, and the fascia-lymphatic interface. Each one plays a unique role, but they are deeply interconnected, what affects one almost always disturbs the others.

The gut lining is responsible for deciding what from your digestive tract is allowed into the bloodstream. In a healthy state, it permits nutrients and blocks pathogens, toxins, and undigested food particles. But when this lining becomes inflamed and porous, what's commonly called "leaky gut," the boundary begins to break down. Substances that don't belong in circulation begin to slip through. The immune system, faced with this unexpected intrusion, becomes reactive and confused. It fires off inflammatory messengers not only locally, but throughout the body, keeping the entire system in a state of quiet alarm.

The blood-brain barrier, equally delicate, is meant to shield the brain from precisely this kind of chaos. It filters what reaches the nervous system, ensuring that only appropriate nutrients and signals pass through. But under chronic stress, whether from toxicity, inflammation, infection, or emotional trauma, this barrier, too, can lose its integrity. When that happens, inflammatory compounds and immune signals that would normally be filtered out reach the brain itself, contributing to neuroinflammation, glial activation, and the progressive disarray of communication between neurons.

The third and often overlooked barrier lies in the fascia and lymphatic system. This isn't a wall in the traditional sense, but a fluid boundary, a circulatory network that clears waste, regulates immune access, and communicates between tissues. When lymph becomes stagnant and fascia grows tight or adhesive, drainage slows. Toxins accumulate. Pressure builds. Communication between cells is distorted, and the body's ability to coordinate repair is compromised.

Together, the failure of these barriers creates a perfect storm: an immune system constantly on edge, a nervous system exposed to molecular threats, and detox pathways that are too burdened to keep up. This is part of what makes ALS terrain so complex. By the time someone reaches visible symptoms, these breakdowns have usually been in motion for years, often silently, without obvious warning.

That's why barrier repair is not the beginning of the healing process, it's the final stage of sealing. Attempting to rebuild the gut or blood-brain barrier before the terrain is ready can be like trying to reseal a dam while the flood is still rising. It won't hold. The body must first be supported in the basics: energy production must be stable, nutrients replenished, toxin inputs reduced, drainage flowing. Only then does the physiology begin to shift from defense into repair.

When that shift occurs, when the body senses that it is no longer under siege, cells begin to regenerate. The gut lining starts renewing itself every few days, as it was always designed to do. The blood-brain barrier tightens, restricting inflammatory signals from crossing into neural tissue. The fascia begins to soften and hydrate, and lymphatic fluid clears more freely. Immune responses become more intelligent, less reactive. And through all of this, the internal world grows quieter.

Barrier repair is not a single event. It is the culmination of everything you've done to stabilize the terrain: feeding it, calming it, clearing it, and now finally, sealing it. When this phase begins in earnest, the body can enter its most profound state of restoration, one in which protection is no longer about hypervigilance, but about coherence, clarity, and calm.

This is the moment when the body stops reacting and starts truly healing. Not because you forced it to, but because you prepared the ground for that possibility to emerge.

Healing the Gut Lining

Of all the internal barriers in the body, the gut lining is perhaps the most foundational. It's also one of the first to break down. Stretching across the entire digestive tract, this single layer of epithelial cells plays a vital role in protecting the bloodstream from unwanted intruders. When intact, it acts as a precise filter, letting nutrients pass through while keeping larger, potentially inflammatory particles out. But when it becomes compromised, which it often does in ALS terrain, the results ripple far beyond digestion.

A damaged gut lining doesn't just cause gastrointestinal discomfort. It allows food proteins, bacterial fragments, mold toxins, and environmental chemicals to "leak" into the bloodstream. The immune system, always vigilant, interprets these leaks as a sign of danger. It responds with alarm signals, launching inflammatory messengers into circulation and priming immune cells into a hyperreactive state. This is one of the ways chronic systemic inflammation begins: not with a single dramatic event, but with the steady seep of unfiltered material across a broken gut wall.

But the gut lining doesn't just protect. It also absorbs. When inflamed or porous, the body's ability to draw in nutrients is diminished. Essential vitamins, minerals, amino acids, and fats, the raw materials needed for nerve repair, mitochondrial energy, and cellular regeneration, may pass through undigested or unabsorbed. In ALS terrain, where the body is already starved at the cellular level, this malabsorption quietly compounds the crisis.

Fortunately, the gut lining is also one of the most regenerative tissues in the body. When given the right inputs, fuel, calm, rhythm, it can begin to rebuild within days. And while there's no magic pill to seal a leaky gut, there is a reliable sequence of support that makes this repair not just possible, but predictable.

The first step is always nourishment, calming, mucosal support through food. Slow-simmered bone broth is one of the most healing tools here. Rich in glycine, proline, and collagen, it provides the amino acids needed to rebuild the connective matrix that holds the intestinal lining together. Teas made from herbs like slippery elm and marshmallow root offer a soothing, coating effect, acting almost like a botanical bandage on inflamed tissue. These mucilaginous herbs don't stimulate or purge, they calm, soften, and shield.

As the digestive system begins to settle, targeted supplements can be layered in. L-glutamine is often the first, because it serves as the primary fuel for the very cells that form the gut lining. When taken consistently, it helps restore the tight junctions that regulate intestinal permeability. Zinc carnosine is another powerful ally, it's been shown to accelerate repair of the epithelial tissue while simultaneously reducing inflammation. For some individuals, high-quality colostrum offers additional support, rich in growth factors and immunoglobulins that help modulate overactive immune responses. However, colostrum must be introduced cautiously, as it's not tolerated by everyone, especially those with dairy sensitivities.

As healing progresses, the signs are often subtle but meaningful. Bloating and gas may decrease. Meals that once triggered fatigue or skin flare-ups become better tolerated. There's a growing sense of calm, not just in the gut, but throughout the body, as inflammation begins to retreat and the immune system no longer sees every bite of food as a threat. Over time, these improvements compound. Nutrient absorption increases. Inflammatory load decreases. And the gut lining, once porous and inflamed, becomes a functional barrier again, resilient, intelligent, and quiet.

Healing the gut isn't a quick fix. It's a process of re-teaching the body that it is safe to receive nourishment, that boundaries can be reestablished, and that repair is not only possible, but already underway.

Rebuilding the Blood-Brain Barrier (BBB)

Your brain is one of the most protected organs in the body, and for good reason. Its delicate neural circuits, intricate signaling systems, and high metabolic demands require a stable internal environment, free from chaotic chemical traffic. That's the job of the blood-brain barrier, or BBB: a microscopic boundary made of tightly connected endothelial cells that line the walls of blood vessels leading into the brain. This barrier doesn't just slow things down; it actively decides what can pass and what must be kept out. Nutrients, oxygen, and glucose are allowed in. Immune triggers, toxins, heavy metals, and pathogens are turned away.

But in ALS and similar terrain collapse conditions, this vital barrier often begins to lose its integrity. When the body is inflamed, depleted, and exposed to chronic stress, whether physical, emotional, or metabolic, the BBB becomes porous. Tight junctions loosen. Protective filtering breaks down. And suddenly, the brain is no longer insulated from the turbulence of the bloodstream. Inflammatory cytokines, immune signals, and even toxicants that would normally be excluded start leaking in. For a nervous system already under pressure, this breach can be devastating.

Neurons are not designed to defend themselves against circulating toxins. They rely on the BBB to do that job. Once that protection fails, microglial cells, the brain's immune sentinels, become hypervigilant. They shift from a calm, watchful state into a reactive, inflammatory mode, releasing signals that further damage neurons and surrounding tissue. This cycle becomes self-sustaining. The more porous the barrier, the more inflamed the brain becomes. And the more inflamed it becomes, the harder it is for the BBB to recover.

But just as the gut lining can regenerate with proper support, so can the blood-brain barrier. The process is not fast, and it cannot be rushed, but it is biologically possible. And it starts with reducing the burden, removing as many inflammatory triggers and metabolic stressors as possible, while introducing the specific nutrients and rhythms that signal the body to begin repair.

Omega-3 fatty acids, especially EPA and DHA, are some of the most important players in this process. These fats are integral to the cell membranes of the brain and the endothelial lining of the BBB itself. They help restore the fluidity, flexibility, and communication between cells that are required to reseal the barrier. They also quiet neuroinflammation, dialing down microglial reactivity and supporting an environment where neurons can focus on signaling rather than defense.

Plant-based compounds called polyphenols offer another layer of protection and repair. Found in foods like blueberries, green tea, and extra virgin olive oil, these molecules have antioxidant and anti-permeability effects. They help stabilize the barrier and prevent further breakdown from oxidative stress. Curcumin, the active compound in turmeric, and resveratrol, found in red grapes and berries, go even further by helping regulate the tight junction proteins that physically hold the BBB together. These compounds don't just scavenge free radicals, they change the way the barrier behaves.

Magnesium also plays a central role in this process, especially in its threonate form. Unlike other forms of magnesium, magnesium threonate is specifically able to cross into the brain and influence both the BBB and the glial cells that maintain its structure. It promotes calm in the nervous system, enhances learning and memory, and supports the physical integrity of this critical boundary.

But rebuilding the blood-brain barrier isn't just about what you take. It's about how you live. Sleep is essential, deep, consistent sleep allows the glymphatic system to clear debris from the brain and gives the BBB time to repair its junctions. Blood sugar regulation is equally important. When glucose levels swing wildly, it creates microvascular damage and oxidative stress, both of which disrupt the barrier. Eating in rhythm, avoiding processed sugars, and prioritizing healthy fats and proteins help maintain the metabolic calm that barrier repair depends on.

As the BBB begins to heal, changes may show up not as dramatic events, but as subtle shifts in clarity and steadiness. You may notice that your thinking feels less foggy, your mood more balanced. The strange heat, fullness, or pressure that sometimes accompanies neuroinflammation may begin to recede. Emotional reactions soften. Sleep deepens, not just in length, but in quality, with more vivid dreams and a sense of actual restoration upon waking.

These are signs that your brain is no longer being constantly triggered from the outside in. They are signs that the barrier, once frayed and overrun, is remembering how to protect you again.

Resetting Fascia and Lymph

There's a part of the healing process that most medical models ignore, not because it's unimportant, but because it doesn't fit easily into the way modern anatomy is taught. It's not an organ. It's not a blood test. It can't be sliced neatly into parts or isolated under a microscope. But without it, healing stalls. This system is the fascia-lymph interface, the soft tissue and fluid network that quietly governs circulation, immune regulation, structural integrity, and trauma storage across the entire body.

Fascia is the connective tissue web that wraps around every muscle, nerve, organ, and vessel. It gives the body shape and coherence, allowing movement without friction and communication without wires. It holds the body together, but it also holds memory. Fascia is sensitive to both physical and emotional trauma. It tightens in response to stress, stiffens in the presence of inflammation, and can remain frozen long after an injury or shock has passed. It is not inert tissue. It responds to your story.

Lymph is the companion system that flows alongside it. It doesn't have a central pump like the heart. Instead, lymphatic fluid moves slowly, powered by breath, muscle movement, and the pulsing of nearby blood vessels. This fluid carries waste, toxins, and immune debris out of tissues and back toward the organs of elimination. It is the drainage highway of the immune system. And just like fascia, it is often congested in ALS terrain.

When fascia is frozen and lymph is stagnant, the terrain becomes sticky and inflamed. Toxins that were mobilized in the gut or cleared from the bloodstream have nowhere to go. Inflammatory signals accumulate around nerves and joints. The immune system stays in clean-up mode, unable to fully reset. You can be doing everything else right, healing the gut, supporting the brain, restoring nutrients, and still feel stuck if this connective system is not moving.

This layer of terrain collapse is often overlooked because it doesn't show up clearly on scans. There's no "lymph panel" in standard bloodwork. But you can feel it. There's a heaviness in the limbs. Puffiness around the face or ankles. A sense of pressure behind the eyes or around the ears. Tenderness in the armpits or groin where lymph nodes sit. Brain fog that feels like a cloud that won't lift. Sometimes there's emotional flatness, too, a frozen, dissociated quality that reflects the body's deeper inability to let go.

But this layer, too, can be restored. Fascia responds to gentle, sustained pressure, through slow movement, craniosacral therapy, manual lymphatic drainage, vibration, or even warm compresses over key nodes. It doesn't need to be forced. In fact, aggressive massage or deep stretching can do more harm than good. What the fascia needs is rhythm, breath, warmth, and permission to release at its own pace. When it begins to soften, lymph flow improves. When lymph begins to move, the terrain starts to clear.

You may notice the signs when this system begins to reset: better tolerance to movement, less internal pressure, clearer skin, less reactivity to environmental triggers, and a new lightness in the body that wasn't there before. Emotional shifts often accompany the physical ones, tears released without warning, memories resurfacing, or a deep feeling of quiet that follows a long-held tension finally letting go.

This is not just detox. This is drainage in its truest form, an unraveling of stagnation, a melting of what has been frozen, and a return to flow. And in terrain healing, flow is everything.

The Goal of This Phase

At this point in the healing journey, much has already been asked of the body, and much has been reclaimed. The terrain is no longer starving. The gut is calmer. Drainage pathways are opening. Nervous system pressure is beginning to lift. But there is still one critical step that must occur before true resilience can take root: the sealing of the internal landscape.

This phase is about closing the leaks, quietly, intentionally, and with deep respect for the body's boundaries. It's not about force or control. It's about honoring the natural architecture of the body and helping it remember how to protect itself again.

In ALS and other terrain collapse conditions, those protective boundaries have been eroded over time. The gut has allowed in what never should have entered. The blood-brain barrier has thinned under the weight of chronic inflammation. The fascia has held tension for too long, and the lymph has carried more waste than it could clear. When these barriers are compromised, the body loses its ability to discern, to decide what belongs and what doesn't. It becomes reactive, inflamed, and overwhelmed.

The purpose of this phase is to reverse that pattern. To reseal the gut so that nutrients are absorbed while threats are excluded. To rebuild the blood-brain barrier so the brain is no longer exposed to every chemical signal or immune disturbance in circulation. To restore the fascia's elasticity and the lymph's quiet rhythm so that detox can proceed without congestion or chaos. This is the phase where the body relearns safety, not just emotionally, but physically, at the cellular and structural level.

Sealing these systems is also about protecting everything you've built so far. The terrain has worked hard to stabilize, to shift out of survival mode. But if detox is introduced too early, if toxins are mobilized while the barriers are still porous, the system can be thrown back into alarm. Inflammation may return. Symptoms may resurface. And the momentum you've cultivated may begin to stall.

That's why this phase matters so deeply. It's a transition from fragility to stability. From reactivity to discernment. From leaking to containment. A sealed terrain doesn't just defend against harm, it becomes intelligent again. It can respond appropriately to stress without overreacting. It can hold nutrients without losing them. It can let go of waste without flooding the system. It can stand strong, not because it is rigid, but because it is coherent.

When this phase is complete, the body no longer feels like it is constantly under siege. There is quiet. There is strength. And most importantly, there is readiness, for the next stage of healing to begin.

Chapter 12: Safe Detox in ALS: A Terrain Approach

Why Detox Must Be Gentle, Sequenced, and Personalized

For many people, the word detox brings to mind something quick and forceful, like a flush, a purge, or a high-dose cleanse meant to "get the bad stuff out fast." That image is not only misleading when it comes to real biology, it can be dangerous, especially in conditions like ALS where the terrain is fragile, inflamed, and deeply under-resourced.

In ALS, the systems that would normally handle detoxification, the liver, kidneys, lymph, and gut, are often already burdened. Mitochondria, which provide the energy required to process and eliminate toxins, are frequently depleted. Immune cells are hyperreactive, quick to interpret any new challenge as a threat. The nervous system is sensitive, inflamed, and vulnerable to overactivation. When toxins are stirred up too quickly in this context, they don't just leave the body, they recirculate. And when they recirculate, they can inflame the brain, stress the mitochondria, and confuse the immune system even further.

This is why aggressive detox strategies, like intense fasting, chelation, or multiple binders at once, can backfire. Rather than bringing relief, they can provoke a reaction that looks and feels like disease progression. These episodes, often called "Herxheimer reactions" or "Herx," can include spikes in inflammation, pain flares, sleep disturbance, increased muscle weakness, or emotional overwhelm. For someone with ALS terrain collapse, these reactions are not just uncomfortable, they can be destabilizing. And they often do more harm than good.

That doesn't mean detox isn't important. It is. In fact, for many people with ALS or similar neurodegenerative conditions, reducing the body's toxic burden is a key part of long-term stabilization. But it has to be done in the right order, at the right pace, and with the right supports in place. Terrain detox is not a single intervention, it's a process. A sequence. A conversation with the body, not a command.

This phase begins only after certain prerequisites are met. The gut must be repaired enough to absorb nutrients and excrete waste without leaking inflammatory triggers into circulation. Drainage pathways, bowels, kidneys, lymph, and sweat, must be open and moving, so that once toxins are mobilized, they actually have a way out. The nervous system must feel safe enough to tolerate a bit of movement and change without sounding the alarm. And most importantly, the terrain must be repleted, fed, hydrated, resourced, and rested, so that detox doesn't drain what little energy the system has left.

When these foundations are in place, detox can begin, but not as a single action. It begins with a signal, a shift. Supporting the body's ability to gently release what no longer serves it. Sometimes that's done through herbs. Sometimes through targeted nutrients, gentle binders, or light sauna therapy. Sometimes it's as simple as increasing hydration, supporting bile flow, or restoring circadian rhythm so the liver can do its work more effectively at night. What matters most is that detox is tailored to you. To your constitution, your symptoms, your rhythms, your capacity. There is no single detox protocol that works for everyone, and there shouldn't be. Your terrain tells the story. And your detox must follow it.

This chapter offers a patient-safe framework for beginning that process. Not a blueprint to rush into, but a roadmap to navigate when the time is right. When the body has been nourished, sealed, and grounded, then, and only then, does it make sense to ask:

What can I begin to release?

Step 1: Reduce Current Exposure

Detox doesn't begin with pulling toxins out of the body. It begins with stopping what's still coming in.

If the body is constantly receiving new exposures, through food, water, air, skin, or medications, it will never have the space or energy to process what's already inside. Trying to push toxins out before cutting off the supply is like trying to bail water from a sinking boat while the leak is still pouring in. The first task is to stop the leak.

In modern life, most of us are surrounded by invisible exposures that accumulate slowly. For someone with ALS terrain collapse, even low levels of these inputs can disrupt healing. That's why reducing toxic burden at the source is not just preventative, it's therapeutic. This step doesn't require perfection. It doesn't demand you change everything overnight. But it does ask you to become aware of the most common sources of incoming toxins, and to begin replacing or removing them in ways that your nervous system and budget can tolerate.

One of the most overlooked sources is cookware. Many nonstick pans, especially older ones, are coated with chemicals like PFOA or PTFE, which release toxic fumes when heated and can leave residues on food. These compounds have been linked to immune dysfunction, hormonal disruption, and even neurological issues. Replacing them with safer alternatives like cast iron, stainless steel, or ceramic is one of the simplest ways to reduce a daily, repeated exposure that affects both the brain and mitochondria.

Dental fillings are another major concern, particularly amalgam fillings that contain mercury. Mercury vapor can leach from these fillings, especially during chewing, grinding, or exposure to heat.

But removing them without proper precautions can be even more dangerous than leaving them in. If amalgam fillings are present, they should never be drilled out by a conventional dentist. Only a trained biological or IAOMT-certified dentist should guide that process. And if those fillings are still in place, it is unsafe to begin chelation or aggressive detox protocols. Mercury must be handled with respect, and timing.

Water is another constant input that many people take for granted. Tap water, even when deemed safe by municipal standards, often contains chlorine, fluoride, lead, pharmaceutical residues, and pesticide runoff. In ALS terrain, where mitochondrial and neurological resilience is already low, these compounds can add to the toxic load daily. Investing in a high-quality filter, such as reverse osmosis or a gravity-based filter like Berkey, can dramatically reduce this exposure. Clean water is not a luxury in this context. It is medicine.

Air quality also matters, especially indoors, where we spend most of our time. Many homes contain mold spores, off-gassing chemicals from furniture and cleaning products, or fine particulate matter from outdoor pollution. Using a HEPA-grade air filter in bedrooms or living spaces, keeping windows open when outdoor air is fresh, and avoiding synthetic air fresheners can help protect a vulnerable respiratory and neurological system. In some cases, remediating hidden mold or improving ventilation makes a profound difference, not just in energy, but in cognition and mood.

What goes on the skin is just as important. The skin is not a passive barrier, it's a porous, living interface with the environment. Lotions, deodorants, soaps, and cosmetics often contain hormone-disrupting chemicals, petroleum derivatives, and artificial fragrances that bypass digestion and enter the bloodstream directly. Switching to unscented, non-toxic products made with simple, plant-based ingredients reduces one more layer of input the liver has to process. These changes may feel small, but they add up daily.

Finally, it's important to take a close look at medications. Many prescription and over-the-counter drugs have known side effects that affect mitochondrial function, liver enzymes, the gut microbiome, or the nervous system. This doesn't mean you should stop taking medications on your own, but it does mean it's worth reviewing them with a practitioner who understands both terrain medicine and pharmacology. In some cases, safer alternatives exist. In others, dosages can be reduced over time. The goal is not to strip away support, but to avoid burdening the body with substances that slow or block the healing process.

Reducing exposure is not glamorous, and it doesn't offer the dramatic promise of a "cleanse." But in terrain medicine, this step is one of the most powerful. When the inflow of toxins slows, the terrain can finally catch its breath. Energy stops going toward constant defense. The immune system becomes less reactive. The nervous system feels less provoked. And the body begins to shift, gently, steadily, toward repair.

This is where detox really begins: not with what you take, but with what you stop taking in.

Step 2: Understand Detox Phases (0–2)

Most people think of detox as a single event, something you do with a product or a protocol. But in reality, detox is a complex, multi-phase process that unfolds in layers. The body doesn't just release toxins all at once. It prepares. It opens exits. It captures and processes waste. And only then, when conditions are safe, does it begin to let go of what's been stored deeper in tissues.

In ALS and similar terrain collapse, understanding this sequence isn't just helpful, it's essential. If you skip steps or push too early, you can overload the system. But when you honor the body's natural phases of detoxification, you reduce risk, avoid overwhelm, and make lasting progress without destabilizing the gains you've already made.

The first phase, sometimes called Phase 0, is what comes before any actual detox begins. This is the foundation phase, and it's the most commonly overlooked. At this point, your focus isn't on pulling toxins out. It's on restoring the body's ability to excrete. That means making sure the bowels are moving regularly, that the lymphatic system is flowing, and that you're consistently hydrated with mineral-rich fluids. If these basic functions aren't in place, any attempt to mobilize toxins from deeper tissues will backfire, because the exits aren't open.

Supporting this phase is simple but powerful. Start with hydration, water alone is not enough. The body needs electrolytes to hold onto water and move it into the cells. Adding sea salt to your drinking water or using herbal teas like nettle, dandelion, or hibiscus can gently support mineral repletion while nourishing the kidneys and liver. Gentle movement, such as walking, stretching, or light bouncing, helps the lymph move, especially when paired with practices like dry brushing or warm castor oil packs over the liver. And perhaps most importantly, sleep and circadian rhythm must be respected. Your detox organs follow a biological clock, and most of their heavy work happens while you sleep. Without that rest, detox simply stalls.

Once these rhythms are established, you can enter Phase 1, which is the drainage and binder phase. This is when the body begins to filter more waste from the blood and digestive system, but only with the help of binders that capture and carry those toxins out.

These binders don't stimulate detox, they simply mop up what's already being processed, preventing it from recirculating and causing inflammation.

The best binders for sensitive terrain are gentle and food-based. Modified citrus pectin, chlorella, and low doses of activated charcoal can all be used selectively. Activated charcoal should be used short-term and never near medication, as it can interfere with absorption. Alongside binders, the liver and gallbladder must be supported to ensure bile flows properly. Bile is one of the primary ways toxins are excreted through the gut, and when it stagnates, detox stops. Herbal bitters like dandelion, artichoke leaf, or gentian can stimulate bile gently. Fiber-rich foods help ensure that once toxins reach the colon, they keep moving. Constipation must be addressed first, if the bowels aren't moving daily, nothing else should proceed.

Only after this groundwork has been laid do you enter Phase 2: gentle mobilization. This is where true detox begins, but only under the right conditions, when the terrain is stable, the exits are clear, and energy reserves are high enough to handle the release of stored toxins from deeper tissues like fat, fascia, and bone.

Mobilization doesn't require pharmaceuticals or extreme cleanses. Food is often enough. Cilantro and parsley, for example, contain compounds that help draw metals from the tissues. Seaweed-based compounds like alginates can bind radioactive elements and heavy metals while supporting thyroid health. Sweating also plays a key role here. Low-temperature saunas, near-infrared (NIR) light, and even simple warm foot soaks can support the skin's role as a detox organ, especially if hydration and mineral intake are consistent. This is also the phase where mitochondrial support becomes especially important, because mobilizing toxins places significant energy demands on the system. Without mitochondrial stability, detox becomes distress, not healing.

Each of these phases builds on the last. They are not linear steps to be rushed through, but interlocking cycles the body can revisit over and over, gently releasing, safely clearing, gradually restoring. This is how true detox works in fragile terrain. Not as a purge, but as a process.

ALS-Specific Cautions: When Not to Chelate

Chelation, the process of pulling heavy metals like mercury, lead, or arsenic out of the body, can be powerful. But in ALS terrain, it is not something to enter lightly. Unlike gentle detoxification through food, binders, or lymph support, chelation forcibly mobilizes metals from deep storage sites in the body and draws them into circulation. If the exits aren't fully open, or if the body is not physiologically prepared to process what's released, this mobilization can cause serious harm.

For individuals with ALS or similar neurodegenerative terrain collapse, the body is often already operating near the edge of overwhelm. Mitochondria are fragile, the nervous system is reactive, and detox organs are underperforming. In this context, chelation can flood the system with more toxicity than it's capable of eliminating. The result isn't healing, it's crisis.

There are clear signs that the body is not yet ready. If your energy levels are still unpredictable, if you crash after meals, feel wired but tired, or can't sustain activity without feeling depleted, this is not the time to chelate. If your bowel movements are irregular, if you're going days without elimination or swinging between constipation and loose stools, your exits are not ready. If your sleep is fragmented, light, restless, or interrupted by early morning waking, your brain is not clearing waste properly. If your emotional state feels volatile, anxious, numb, or dysregulated, the nervous system is still in defense mode, and detox will likely feel like an assault.

Another non-negotiable rule: do not begin any chelation protocol if you still have mercury amalgam fillings in your mouth. These fillings continue to release vaporized mercury every time you eat, chew, or drink something warm. Chelating with fillings in place can draw even more mercury into circulation, worsening neurological damage. Fillings must be removed safely, by a trained biological dentist who uses proper isolation techniques, and only once the body has been prepared to handle the shift.

Even with all the right preparation, it's possible to over-mobilize. When that happens, the warning signs can be subtle at first, then rapidly escalate. You may feel a rise in muscle twitching, new waves of weakness, or sudden spikes of panic that seem disconnected from your thoughts. Some people describe a sensation of head pressure, heat, or what they call a "burning brain" feeling. Skin may flare with rashes or itching. Sleep may vanish. You might feel like you're regressing, or even experiencing a worsening of your disease. This is not a sign that "detox is working." It's a sign that your system is overwhelmed.

If any of these symptoms occur, stop the mobilization immediately. That means stopping chelating agents, detox-stimulating herbs, or sauna therapy. Return to basics: hydration, mineral repletion, and binders. Increase rest. Increase warmth and emotional safety. Rebuild drainage before even considering trying again. Detox in ALS terrain must follow the body's pace, not our will.

Chelation may have a place in long-term recovery, especially when metals are clearly driving neurological damage. But only when the foundation is strong, the exits are flowing, and the terrain is truly ready. The goal isn't just to remove toxins, it's to do so in a way that protects, not provokes, the nervous system. In fragile terrain, the how and when matter just as much as the what.

Supportive Cofactors That Make Detox Safer

Detox is not simply about getting toxins out. It's about how well the body can handle what's being released, and that depends heavily on whether the right biochemical supports are in place. In ALS terrain, where energy is limited and the nervous system is easily overwhelmed, these supportive cofactors are what make the difference between a healing process and a setback. They don't accelerate detox, they stabilize it. They protect mitochondria, soothe the brain, and make sure the liver has what it needs to process toxins without becoming overburdened.

At the center of this support system is glutathione, often referred to as the body's "master antioxidant." Glutathione is essential for protecting cells, especially neurons and mitochondria, from oxidative stress. It also plays a central role in Phase II liver detoxification, the step where toxins are neutralized and made water-soluble so they can be safely excreted. But in chronic illness terrain, glutathione is often depleted. To restore it, some people use liposomal glutathione directly, while others prefer to support the body's own production of it through precursors like N-acetylcysteine, or NAC.

NAC does more than just raise glutathione. It also breaks down mucus and biofilms, protective layers that pathogens and toxins can hide behind in the gut and respiratory tract. By softening these barriers, NAC allows the immune system and detox organs to access and process long-standing debris more effectively. It's a gentle way to support terrain without pushing it.

Magnesium is another essential cofactor that's often undervalued during detox. It doesn't just relax muscles or improve sleep, it plays a direct role in the enzyme systems that govern Phase II detoxification. Without adequate magnesium, these enzymes can stall, causing partially processed toxins to accumulate in the system. In ALS terrain, where muscle tension, cramping, and spasms are common, magnesium also helps calm neuromuscular overactivity. The best forms, such as glycinate or malate, are easy on the digestive system and well absorbed.

B vitamins are critical players in this phase, particularly B1 (thiamine), B6 (as P5P), B12 (as methyl- or hydroxycobalamin), and folate (as methylfolate or folinic acid). These nutrients don't just support energy, they are required for methylation, the biochemical pathway that helps clear toxins from the body and repair damaged neurons. Without sufficient B vitamins, especially in bioavailable forms, the nervous system struggles to maintain resilience during detox, and recovery can stall.

The liver and bile system also need support. As toxins are processed, they are pushed into bile to be sent into the intestines for removal. But if bile is sluggish or thick, toxins get recycled instead of released. Simple, food-based supports can make a significant difference here. Bitter herbs like dandelion root, gentian, or artichoke leaf can gently stimulate bile flow. Foods like beets and lemons help thin the bile and improve circulation through the liver. Phosphatidylcholine, a key component of cell membranes, also supports bile formation and helps repair liver tissue.

Sweating is another important but often underused detox pathway. The skin is a vast excretory organ, and stimulating it in low-impact ways can gently unload the toxic burden from deeper systems. Near-infrared (NIR) light, low-heat saunas, foot soaks, and even warm compresses applied over key lymphatic areas can all encourage release through the skin. For those who can't tolerate heat or prolonged sweating, rhythmic movement, such as stretching, fascia rolling, or walking, can stimulate sweat and lymph without triggering exhaustion.

These cofactors are not accessories, they are safeguards. They ensure that detox doesn't push too far, too fast. They create a biochemical safety net beneath the process, giving the body the resources it needs to metabolize and release without triggering fear, inflammation, or fatigue.

In terrain-based healing, every layer of support matters. The goal isn't to detox aggressively, it's to detox intelligently. And that begins by listening to the body, strengthening its core systems, and making sure the tools used are as gentle and wise as the process itself.

Signs You Are Detoxing at the Right Pace

One of the most important truths in terrain healing is that detox should not feel like a crisis. Despite what popular culture and online forums might suggest, intense detox reactions are not a badge of honor. They are often a sign that the body has been pushed too far, too fast.

True detox, especially in fragile terrain like ALS, should feel like a gradual unfolding. The body shouldn't be thrown into chaos. It should feel steadier. Quieter. More supported. The signs of a well-paced detox are subtle but clear, and they speak not through dramatic flare-ups, but through stability.

You may begin to notice that sleep, which may have been fragmented or light, becomes deeper. You wake with less mental fog and feel more rested, even if your sleep duration hasn't changed. Your energy may become more even throughout the day, not in bursts followed by crashes, but in gentle waves that allow you to move and rest without strain. Bowel movements, once irregular or incomplete, begin to follow a predictable rhythm. This isn't just a sign of digestive repair, it's proof that toxins are being eliminated instead of recirculated.

Mentally, clarity starts to return. You might find it easier to organize your thoughts or make decisions that used to feel overwhelming. Memory improves, not dramatically all at once, but in glimmers. Words come a little easier. Emotional resilience follows. You may still feel sadness, grief, or frustration, but your reactions become softer, more measured. Your nervous system no longer feels as raw or as close to the edge.

Your skin, often one of the first places detox distress shows up, begins to shift too. Where there was dullness or reactivity, you may notice a slight glow returning, color, softness, a sense that your body is clearing from the inside out. Most importantly, there is no new spike in neurological symptoms. Twitching doesn't intensify. Weakness doesn't deepen. There's no sense of increased agitation, head pressure, or cognitive disruption. Instead, your symptoms either remain stable or begin to gently improve.

These are the signs that detox is aligned with your terrain's capacity. That your exits are open, your supports are in place, and your body is no longer drowning in inputs. You're not just flushing toxins, you're creating space for healing to unfold without fear.

If the terrain feels calmer, clearer, and more coherent, you're on the right path. That's what detox done well should feel like.

Chapter 13: Addressing Hidden Infections: A Terrain Strategy

Why Hidden Infections Matter in ALS Terrain

Not all threats to the body are loud or obvious. Some of the most damaging are quiet, hidden below the surface, evading detection while draining the terrain year after year. These are the stealth infections: microbes that don't cause dramatic fevers or acute illness, but instead linger in tissues, hijack resources, and confuse the immune system until the terrain begins to break down.

In ALS and other chronic neurodegenerative conditions, these infections often go undiagnosed, not because they're rare, but because they're skilled at hiding. They may not show up in standard bloodwork. They may not create a single clear symptom that points to them directly. But if you know how to listen to the terrain, you can often recognize their fingerprint.

Stealth pathogens operate differently from the microbes we associate with short-term illness. They burrow deep into tissues, into the gut lining, the nervous system, the lymph nodes, and even inside the mitochondria themselves. They create biofilms, protective structures that shield them from immune surveillance and antibiotics. They communicate with one another chemically, creating colonies that shift and adapt in response to your biology. Some of them, like Borrelia (Lyme), Bartonella, Babesia, Mycoplasma, Epstein-Barr virus, HHV-6, or intestinal parasites, are commonly found in those with ALS-like terrain, even when standard labs say everything is "normal."

Why does this matter? Because these organisms place enormous stress on the terrain. They drain energy at the cellular level by disrupting mitochondrial function. They trigger chronic immune activation, low-grade, often silent, but relentless. They interfere with the gut-brain axis, throwing off vagal tone, mood, digestion, and neurological balance. And they send false signals that confuse the immune system, sometimes leading to autoimmunity or neuroinflammatory states that seem to come out of nowhere.

In terrain collapse, where energy and resilience are already compromised, these infections create an invisible burden. The immune system can't fully clear them, but it also can't fully ignore them. So it stays activated, burning through resources, mistaking friend for foe, and misfiring into the nervous system itself. Over time, this constant low-level warfare erodes the integrity of the terrain. What began as fatigue, digestive irregularity, or sensitivity becomes something much more complex.

But there is hope. These infections are not invincible. While they may resist direct attack, they are highly sensitive to the state of the terrain. When the gut is sealed, when lymph is flowing, when the mitochondria are supported and the immune system is guided rather than suppressed, stealth pathogens lose their advantage. They can no longer hide as effectively. Their biofilms weaken. Their signaling patterns become disrupted. And most importantly, your body can begin to regain control.

The goal of this chapter is not to fear these infections, but to understand them. To recognize their patterns, support the systems they target, and create an environment where they can no longer thrive. Testing can be helpful, but symptoms and terrain history often tell a deeper truth. If you've done the work to stabilize and seal the terrain, this is the next step: addressing the invisible organisms that have kept the body locked in defense mode for far too long.

Symptom-Based Recognition of Stealth Pathogens

In an ideal world, lab tests would clearly reveal the root causes of complex illness. But in the case of stealth infections, the body often tells a clearer story than the lab. These organisms are experts at evading detection, they hide inside cells, form biofilms, or cycle between active and dormant phases that make their footprints hard to track with conventional diagnostics. As a result, many people struggling with these infections are told their tests are "normal," even when their bodies are clearly signaling otherwise.

This is where terrain-based medicine offers something different: pattern recognition. By listening to the rhythm of symptoms, the timing of flares, and the subtle clues the body offers, we can begin to map the presence of hidden pathogens, even without a perfect test. The following patterns aren't meant to replace clinical diagnosis. But they can help guide support strategies and give meaning to symptoms that are often dismissed.

Viral Reactivation (EBV, HHV-6, CMV)

Certain viruses, once contracted, never fully leave the body. Instead, they go dormant, hidden in tissues, waiting for a moment of vulnerability. In ALS terrain, where the immune system is under strain, these viruses can reactivate quietly and cyclically. Epstein-Barr virus (EBV), human herpesvirus 6 (HHV-6), and cytomegalovirus (CMV) are some of the most common culprits.

People often describe waves of unexplained fatigue that come and go without clear cause. There may be subtle flu-like symptoms, soreness behind the eyes, muscle heaviness, or low-grade fever without an actual cold. Depression may deepen during these times, and a heaviness sets in that sleep doesn't fully relieve. Neck tension, especially around the lymph nodes, or tenderness near the spleen may appear during a flare. Cold sores or shingles may surface, especially after emotional stress or physical overexertion. These aren't coincidences, they're signs the immune system is dancing with viral reactivation.

Mycoplasma or Intracellular Bacteria

Some infections don't live in the blood or on the skin, they burrow deep inside the cells themselves. Mycoplasma, Chlamydia pneumoniae, and other intracellular bacteria are notorious for this. They provoke constant low-grade inflammation that doesn't fully resolve, leading to a vague but relentless sense of illness.

The terrain picture often includes persistent fatigue, joint or muscle pain that migrates or intensifies with activity, and an unusual sensation known as "air hunger", feeling like you can't get a satisfying breath, even when your lungs are clear. This isn't just anxiety. It's a biochemical disturbance caused by impaired mitochondrial energy and oxygen handling. Cognitive symptoms may worsen with physical exertion, a hallmark of post-exertional malaise. These infections drain energy and sabotage the body's ability to recover from even mild stressors.

Lyme (Borrelia) and Co-Infections (Bartonella, Babesia)

Tick-borne infections like Lyme disease and its co-infections are especially complex, often masquerading as other conditions. In ALS terrain, they may contribute to flares of neurological symptoms, shifting sensitivities, or bizarre sensations that seem to move from one body part to another.

Wandering pain, especially in joints, nerves, or the jaw, is a key clue. Sensory sensitivity may increase, including intolerance to sound, light, temperature changes, or even electromagnetic fields (EMFs). These are signs that the peripheral and central nervous systems are inflamed or dysregulated. Some people notice that symptoms worsen overnight, particularly around 3 a.m., disrupting sleep and leaving them with a strange morning "buzzing" or electric feeling. Unlike typical infections, which follow a linear course, these pathogens fluctuate unpredictably, another sign of stealth.

Gut-Driven Immune Confusion (Candida, Parasites)

Not all stealth pathogens are viruses or bacteria. The gut itself can harbor yeast overgrowth (like Candida albicans) or parasites that create chronic immune confusion. These organisms generate toxins, disrupt digestion, and provoke allergic or inflammatory responses that ripple throughout the body.

The clues are often digestive and behavioral. There may be intense sugar cravings or a strong desire for bread, alcohol, or starch, foods that feed yeast and certain parasites. Bloating, gas, or loose stools may accompany these cravings, followed by mood swings or a sense of internal agitation. Skin itching, especially in the ears, scalp, or around the anus, is another hallmark. Histamine sensitivity may increase, showing up as rashes, flushing, or food reactions. Symptoms often cycle in a predictable pattern, worsening after certain foods or around the full moon, when many parasites become more active.

Stealth infections speak in patterns. They don't always scream, they whisper. But if you know how to listen, you can begin to understand which systems are involved, and what kind of support may be needed. The next step is not to attack them head-on, but to shift the terrain so that they no longer have control.

Natural Antimicrobials for Terrain-Sensitive Use

When it comes to treating hidden infections in fragile terrain, gentleness and intelligence must come before intensity. The conventional approach to chronic infection often mirrors warfare: antibiotics, antivirals, and antifungals launched like missiles, with little regard for the body's collateral damage. But terrain-based healing takes a different view. Rather than focusing solely on

139

"killing" pathogens, we look to shift the ecosystem, making the internal environment less hospitable to stealth organisms while strengthening the body's natural defenses.

Natural antimicrobials, when chosen and used carefully, can support this strategy beautifully. They're often gentler than pharmaceuticals, yet still potent when aligned with the body's rhythms. They don't suppress immunity, they guide it. Many of these herbs and compounds offer additional benefits, like calming inflammation, protecting mitochondria, or soothing the gut lining. But timing and dosing matter. In terrain that's easily overwhelmed, these remedies must be introduced slowly, often in rotation or pulses, with a careful eye on symptom feedback.

Antivirals

Lemon balm is one of the most terrain-friendly antivirals available. Known botanically as Melissa officinalis, it has a long history of use against herpes family viruses like Epstein-Barr (EBV) and HHV-6. But its true gift is its dual action: it's not just antiviral, it's calming. It soothes the nervous system, eases tension, and supports better sleep, making it especially helpful when viral flares provoke anxiety or restlessness.

Lomatium is a much stronger plant. It acts broadly against many viruses, but its power comes with a caution, it must be pulsed (used for short stretches, then paused) and introduced slowly. Some people react to it with a skin rash or immune flare, especially if detox pathways aren't clear. When tolerated, it can be a game-changer for persistent viral load, but it requires respect.

Licorice root, particularly in its deglycyrrhizinated form (DGL), is gentle and versatile. It's often used to soothe the gut lining, but it also helps balance cortisol and support immune function in people who are chronically depleted. In viral terrain, especially when stress and fatigue are intertwined, licorice can help the body find its footing again.

Monolaurin is a compound derived from coconut that targets enveloped viruses, including EBV, CMV, and some flu viruses. It works by disrupting the viral envelope, the coating that helps viruses invade host cells. Monolaurin is generally well tolerated, though like any antimicrobial, it may provoke temporary die-off symptoms if introduced too quickly.

Antibacterials

Andrographis is a powerful herbal immune stimulant, often used in both bacterial and viral infections. It shines in cases where the immune system needs a strategic nudge rather than full activation. It's particularly helpful in Lyme and co-infection patterns, but should be introduced cautiously in those with high inflammation, as it may provoke a short-term immune flare.

Cat's claw (Uncaria tomentosa) offers broad-spectrum antibacterial support while also reducing inflammation and protecting the blood-brain barrier. It's used widely in terrain-sensitive Lyme protocols, especially where neurological symptoms or cognitive fog are present. Unlike many herbs, it seems to both clear pathogens and calm the system at the same time.

Cryptolepis is a strikingly potent herb with antimalarial properties and activity against bacteria, viruses, and parasites. It has a long traditional use in African and Chinese medicine and is now gaining attention for its effectiveness in Lyme, Babesia, and Mycoplasma terrain. Because of its strength, it should be introduced slowly and usually not used continuously for long periods without practitioner oversight.

Garlic, especially in aged extract form, offers a gentle but broad-spectrum antimicrobial effect. It's antibacterial, antifungal, antiparasitic, and supports bile flow, making it a great ally for gut-driven infection terrain. For those who tolerate it well, whole garlic (raw or lightly cooked) can be used daily to support immune resilience and microbial balance.

Biofilm Disruptors

Pathogens that hide in chronic illness don't float freely in the bloodstream. They form protective communities called biofilms, complex networks made of proteins, sugars, and fats that shield them from immune detection and antimicrobial agents. Breaking through these structures is essential, and certain compounds help make that possible.

Serrapeptase is a proteolytic enzyme originally derived from silkworms. It helps break down the protein scaffolding that holds biofilms together, allowing the immune system and antimicrobials to access hidden organisms. It's often used in pulsed fashion and can also help with inflammation and scar tissue.

NAC (N-acetylcysteine) is well-known for supporting glutathione production, but it also works as a biofilm disruptor. It thins mucus, breaks apart microbial shield layers, and softens congestion, whether in the lungs, sinuses, or gut. Its dual action makes it especially useful when detox and infection overlap.

Curcumin, the active compound in turmeric, is not only a powerful anti-inflammatory, it also penetrates biofilms and reduces immune overactivation. It supports cognitive clarity, calms gut inflammation, and modulates microglial activity in the brain. In chronic infection terrain, curcumin often serves as a bridge, allowing the immune system to engage pathogens without overreacting.

Used wisely, these tools help shift the terrain back into balance. They don't force, they assist. They don't override, they guide. This is the heart of terrain-based infection support: working with the body, not against it.

How to Pulse and Sequence Antimicrobials Safely

Introducing antimicrobials, whether herbs, enzymes, or supplements, is not just about choosing the right substance. It's about timing, pacing, and listening. In a sensitive terrain, especially one affected by ALS, the way you take something is often more important than what you take.

Natural antimicrobials may seem harmless compared to pharmaceuticals, but they are still powerful agents. When introduced too early or in the wrong sequence, they can overwhelm a fragile system. Even herbs that are considered "gentle" can provoke strong reactions in a body that's already working overtime to stabilize inflammation, repair tissues, and clear metabolic waste.

The first rule is this: do not begin antimicrobial therapy until the body is ready. This means the gut lining has been partially sealed, basic drainage pathways, like bowel movements, lymph flow, and urination, are functioning consistently, and the person has reached a level of relative energy stability. If sleep is shallow or chaotic, if emotions are still swinging between anxiety and shutdown, or if the digestive system is reactive to food, it's too soon. Start with terrain support. Come back to this step later.

Once the foundation is solid, you can begin using a pulsing strategy. Pulsing means using antimicrobials for short bursts, typically three to five days, followed by a rest period of two to three days. This approach mimics natural rhythms and allows the body to process what's being released without becoming overwhelmed. During the off days, the immune system recalibrates, drainage continues, and mitochondria catch their breath.

These pauses are critical. They're not a sign of weakness, they're a sign of wisdom. If you notice new fatigue, headaches, rashes, pain flares, or a wave of emotional unease during an antimicrobial pulse, those are signs the body is working hard to clear debris. You may need to slow down, reduce the dose, or add more support for detoxification. Never push through symptoms in hopes of killing off more pathogens. In terrain medicine, the goal is not eradication, it's balance.

Sequencing also matters. In general, antivirals are the safest place to start. They tend to provoke fewer die-off reactions, and many have a calming effect on the nervous system. Once those are tolerated, antibacterial herbs, such as cat's claw, cryptolepis, or garlic, can be layered in gradually. These are more likely to provoke immune flares or detox reactions, so they should be introduced with even greater caution.

Biofilm disruptors should come last. These tools expose hidden infections by breaking down their protective shields. That makes them incredibly effective, but also risky if the terrain is not fully prepared. Only introduce biofilm agents once binders are in place and consistently tolerated, and once the body is eliminating daily through stool, urine, sweat, and breath. Otherwise, the pathogens released from their hiding places may flood the system with toxins faster than it can cope.

Throughout all antimicrobial phases, cellular protection and excretion support must continue. Binders like citrus pectin, chlorella, or activated charcoal can help mop up what's being released. Hydration and bile-stimulating herbs (like bitters or lemon water) keep the liver and gallbladder flowing. Magnesium helps calm spasms, nerve agitation, and muscle tightness that can follow microbial die-off. And glutathione or its precursors like

NAC protect mitochondria and prevent oxidative stress as the body detoxifies.

This is not a race. Some people pulse one herb at a time, others rotate families of herbs on a weekly or monthly basis. What matters most is that the body remains stable as the terrain is cleared. If there is clarity, calmness, and improvement, you're on the right track. If things begin to feel chaotic or overwhelming, that's a cue to pause, not push.

In healing chronic infection, force doesn't equal progress. Alignment does. When you work with the body's rhythm, when you respect the timing, the feedback, and the signals, antimicrobials become allies, not invaders. And the terrain becomes less a battleground and more a place where balance can be restored.

Terrain-Specific Cautions

When working with natural antimicrobials in fragile terrain, caution is not a sign of fear, it's a form of respect. The ALS body is not a blank canvas. It is a complex, sensitized ecosystem that has already endured years of oxidative stress, immune confusion, and energy depletion. It has likely compensated in every way it can. So before introducing any agents that might stir up hidden infections, we must pause and ask: Is the body ready for this step?

There are specific red flags that tell us when the terrain is not yet prepared for antimicrobial intervention. If any of these are present, it's important to delay and focus instead on foundational support.

First, check elimination. If you are constipated, not sweating at all, or urinating infrequently, toxins have nowhere to go. Starting antimicrobials in this state is like kicking up dust in a sealed room, it will only settle back into sensitive tissues, including the brain and nerves. Ensure bowel movements are happening daily, sweat is gently encouraged (even if only through warm compresses or movement), and the lymph system is flowing before mobilizing anything.

Second, look at tolerance. If your body is still reacting to basic foods or supplements, it's not ready for deeper clearing. You must first reach a point where your digestion is relatively calm, your sleep is restorative, and your system can handle simple inputs without flaring. This shows the immune system is grounded enough to engage with new information, like herbs, without going into alarm.

Third, assess emotional stability. If you're in a place of panic, despair, or deep overwhelm, even a small shift in chemistry can trigger a disproportionate reaction. Antimicrobials can stir emotional debris stored in fascia or the brainstem. If sleep is highly disrupted or you're feeling fragile emotionally, it's better to wait until nervous system safety is more firmly in place.

Finally, consider mold exposure. If you are still living or working in an environment with active mold, antimicrobial therapy will likely backfire. Mold toxins suppress the immune system, damage mitochondria, and destabilize terrain. You cannot out-supplement ongoing exposure. Address the environment first.

Even if you feel ready, it's essential to recognize the early signs of a Herxheimer reaction, also known as die-off. This happens when the body is flooded with microbial waste products faster than it can eliminate them. Some of the most common signs include a sudden spike in neurological symptoms (increased twitching, tremors, or heaviness), emotional instability (panic, dread, or unprovoked irritability), head pressure, joint pain, rashes, or a mysterious low-grade fever. These symptoms are your body's way of saying: slow down.

If any of these arise during a pulse or shortly after starting a new herb, stop antimicrobial therapy immediately. Don't push through. Instead, increase hydration. Take binders to mop up circulating toxins. Support the lymph with dry brushing, castor oil packs, gentle stretching, or warm baths. Prioritize rest and sleep. Let your system settle fully before considering a return.

And when you do return, do so with less intensity, fewer herbs, lower doses, shorter pulses. The terrain remembers what overwhelmed it. It also remembers what helped it feel safe again.

This process is not linear. It's layered. The goal is not to race toward "killing off" pathogens, it's to move in harmony with the body's capacity to respond, eliminate, and repair. Caution isn't just appropriate here. It's essential.

Encouragement for This Phase

It's easy to fall into the mindset that hidden infections must be fought, conquered, or eradicated. The language of war, "killing pathogens," "attacking biofilms," "eliminating invaders", is common in chronic illness spaces. But this chapter, like the terrain itself, offers a different path forward.

The goal here is not to "kill everything." It is to restore rhythm. To rebalance the ecosystem that has been disrupted, and to support the body in returning to its natural intelligence. Pathogens, especially the stealth ones that linger in ALS terrain, only thrive when the body is out of sync. They take advantage of low energy, broken barriers, and misfiring signals. But when the terrain is nourished, hydrated, and safe, these organisms lose their grip.

Healing from infection in this model is not about domination. It is about making the terrain inhospitable to dysfunction, and doing so in a way that does not cause further harm. This means resisting the urge to push aggressively, even when fear or frustration arises.

It means trusting your pacing and allowing your body to lead.

And perhaps most importantly, it means not retraumatizing the nervous system in the name of progress. Many people with ALS terrain have experienced years of medical trauma, misdiagnosis, or bodily betrayal. So pushing too hard, too fast can easily trigger collapse. This phase must be approached with gentleness, not force. With curiosity, not control. With permission to pause whenever your body says it needs rest.

You are not broken. You are not overrun. Your body is doing the best it can to survive in the face of invisible burdens. The infections that linger are not your fault. And you do not need to conquer them all at once to make meaningful progress.

Instead of fighting, think of this phase as unfreezing, releasing what has been locked up, both biologically and emotionally. Clearing stagnation. Softening hypervigilance. Making space for vitality to return.

There is no perfect protocol. But there is a wise, listening relationship you can build with your terrain. And from that place, healing becomes not just possible, but inevitable.

Chapter 14: Build Your Personalized Terrain Map

Terrain Healing Isn't One-Size-Fits-All

It's tempting to want a step-by-step plan, something clear, specific, and universal. Especially in the face of a condition as complex and overwhelming as ALS, many people crave structure: Just tell me what to do and I'll do it. But the truth is, healing terrain isn't a checklist, it's a relationship. And like all relationships, it needs to be tailored to the individual.

While ALS often follows a recognizable trajectory, gut dysfunction, mitochondrial collapse, neuroinflammation, immune misfiring, the sequence and intensity of those breakdowns vary from person to person. Some people experience rapid progression; others plateau. Some struggle most with movement, others with speech, digestion, or emotional regulation. The "what" may look similar, but the "how" and "when" of healing will always be personal.

That's why your terrain map must start with you, not someone else's story, not a rigid protocol, and not an abstract theory. Your path forward needs to honor your real-time, lived reality. What are your current symptoms, not past ones or imagined future ones? How much energy do you have available each day, honestly? What is your emotional state, are you feeling safe, grounded, resourced enough to take on more, or already near your edge? Do you have people around you who can help? What can you afford in terms of time, energy, and money? These are not limitations, they are the raw materials of your healing architecture.

This chapter is about helping you build scaffolding, not a cage. A terrain map that bends and flexes as you do. One that respects setbacks without labeling them failure, and recognizes small wins as the foundational bricks of long-term change.

You are not meant to fit into a program. A program must respond to you, your body, your rhythm, your inner compass. Terrain healing is not a destination, but a direction. And the map you build now will help you keep moving forward, even when the path twists or narrows.

This is your terrain. And no one knows it more intimately than you.

Start Exactly Where You Are

One of the greatest misconceptions about healing is the belief that we must begin from some ideal starting line, well-resourced, symptom-free, perfectly prepared. But terrain healing meets you exactly where you are. Not where you wishyou were. Not where someone else thinks you should be. And certainly not where a protocol assumes you are.

There is no perfect place to begin. There is only your terrain, in its current expression. That is your foundation.

Instead of looking for the "right" entry point, look for the place that is most ready, most urgent, or most accessibletoday. Begin with what's loudest, or what's most willing. That might be the symptom that's screaming for attention, like relentless insomnia, blood sugar crashes, or chronic dehydration. Stabilizing one of these core rhythms can unlock progress across the whole system.

Or you might start with the most obvious block in your terrain, something that keeps creating downstream chaos. If you're not pooping regularly, for example, no amount of detox support will help. If chronic stress is hijacking your nervous system daily, gut healing and immune balance will stay out of reach. If you're barely eating protein, your body won't have the raw materials it needs to rebuild tissues or support mitochondria.

In some cases, the best place to begin is the easiest available win, the low-hanging fruit. That could be switching your drinking water to a cleaner source, adding mineral-rich sea salt to meals, or removing one food you know causes discomfort. These small changes may seem too simple, but they build trust. They signal safety. They prove to your body that support is real and consistent. And often, they open doors to deeper work.

You can also begin with the system that feels the most depleted. If fatigue is crushing or your muscles don't recover from basic movement, mitochondrial repletion may need to come first. If you feel emotionally flat or wired but exhausted, nervous system support may be your entry point. If your digestion feels inflamed and reactive, the gut may be the gateway.

There is no shame in beginning small. There is wisdom in beginning true. When you meet your body where it actually is, not where you think it should be, you build healing momentum that's sustainable.

This is not about fixing everything at once. It's about taking the next step that your body says "yes" to.

Divide Your Map into Phases (Layered Terrain Model)

Trying to do everything at once is one of the fastest ways to overwhelm a fragile body. Especially in a condition like ALS, where energy is precious and systems are interlinked, healing must happen in phases. Each layer builds upon the previous one. Each step must be earned, not assumed. And the decision to move forward should come from clear, embodied feedback, not urgency, fear, or pressure.

This layered terrain model helps you structure your healing into manageable phases. But more importantly, it gives you a way to listen to your body at every stage. You don't move on because you've hit a deadline or completed a checklist. You move forward because your body says, "I'm ready."

Phase 1: Stabilize and Replete

This is the foundation. Before any repair, detox, or clearing can happen, your body needs basic physiological rhythms restored. Blood sugar must be steady. Sleep must be restorative. Bowel movements must be daily and easy. Electrolytes must be balanced. These aren't luxuries, they are the pillars of a responsive, self-healing terrain.

This phase includes mineral repletion (magnesium, potassium, trace minerals), adrenal supports like vitamin C and glycine, and grounding foods like soups, cooked vegetables, healthy fats, and soft proteins like egg yolks. It's about calm nourishment, not restriction.

How you'll know you're ready to move forward:
Energy becomes more stable throughout the day. You recover better from small efforts. You notice less reactivity to foods or stimuli. Your elimination and sleep follow a solid rhythm. There's a felt sense of having more in reserve.

Phase 2: Seal and Calm the Gut–Brain Axis

With the body more stable, attention turns to the core signaling highway between the gut and the brain. When this connection is inflamed or leaking, everything else becomes distorted, immunity, cognition, and emotional resilience. This phase focuses on healing the gut lining, calming the immune system, and restoring the nervous system's sense of safety.

Here, you may remove inflammatory triggers like gluten, dairy, soy, corn, yeast, or even nightshades and eggs if sensitivity is suspected. You'll bring in gut-repair supports like glutamine, colostrum, and zinc carnosine. Just as importantly, you'll use warm, grounding food and somatic tools to reinforce nervous system calm, because the gut cannot heal in a fight-or-flight state.

Signals you're ready to advance:
Bloating, rashes, or histamine flares begin to lessen. Your mood and mental clarity stabilize. You find you tolerate foods and supplements more easily. Emotional swings soften. Inflammation feels more manageable.

Phase 3: Drain and Detox Safely

Now that the terrain has a stronger boundary and a calmer center, you can begin opening the exits, supporting the body's ability to release what it no longer needs. This is not the time for aggressive detox or chelation. It is a time for drainage: supporting the kidneys, liver, lymph, skin, bowels, and lungs so they can function as natural elimination channels.

Start with hydration enriched with sea salt and lemon. Use castor oil packs, dry brushing, gentle movement, and liver bitters. Introduce binders like citrus pectin or chlorella, but only once bowel movements are regular and daily. At this point, mitochondrial protectors like glutathione, NAC, and CoQ10 are essential, as detox will stir up oxidative stress.

ALS-specific caution:
Chelation and toxin mobilization should never be attempted until the terrain is stable, physically, emotionally, and environmentally. If you still have mercury fillings, do not begin chelation. If your sleep, mood, or energy are highly unstable, focus instead on rest and drainage. Detox is only medicine if the body is ready.

Phase 4: Address Pathogens and Infections (Optional Timing)

Not everyone with ALS terrain will need to engage this phase directly. But if stealth infections are part of your picture, if symptoms point toward reactivated viruses, intracellular bacteria, or chronic gut imbalances, this is the time to gently begin addressing them.

Use pulsed herbal antimicrobials like monolaurin, cat's claw, or cryptolepis. If biofilms are suspected, consider tools like NAC or serrapeptase, but only after drainage and binder support is well established. You are not trying to kill everything. You are nudging the terrain back into balance, step by step.

How to know it's time:
Your body is eliminating clearly. Your sleep and mood are steady. You can tolerate mild provocation (e.g., detox teas, antimicrobial foods) without crashing. You feel more curious than afraid about this work.

Phase 5: Reconnect and Regenerate

This is where deep healing happens, not just biologically, but at the level of rhythm, identity, and coherence. After the body is no longer on fire, it can begin to rebuild. Neuroplasticity returns. The nervous system can release stored trauma. Brain-body communication improves. Energy becomes creative, not just survival-based.

This is the phase for limbic retraining tools like DNRS or Primal Trust, somatic therapies that reconnect you to safety, and breathwork that restores vagal tone. This is where peptides or herbs that promote neuroregeneration, like lion's mane, bacopa, and BDNF-enhancing nutrients, can be introduced. Movement and vocalization practices help rewire the brain and integrate new patterns of function.

This phase does not mark "the end." It simply reflects a new relationship with your terrain, one based not on symptom suppression or protocol following, but on deep repair and emerging vitality.

Use Symptoms as Your Compass

Your body speaks in signals, not always in words, but in patterns, shifts, and sensations. It tells you when something is helping, when something is too much, and when something needs to pause. The key to personalized terrain healing is learning how to listen, not with anxiety, but with grounded curiosity.

This is not about becoming hypervigilant or tracking every detail with a microscope. It's about noticing the broad strokes. Are you moving in the direction of stability, or strain? Of rhythm, or chaos? Symptoms aren't random, they're information. And in terrain work, they become your compass.

Let's start with the green lights, the signs that your body is saying "yes." These might include a steadier energy curve throughout the day, more predictable bowel movements, a calmer emotional baseline, or the simple return of hunger cues or deeper sleep. You may find yourself reacting less intensely to food, people, or stress. These are all signals that your interventions are aligned with what your terrain needs.

Then there are the yellow lights. These don't mean you're doing harm, they just signal that your body is asking for awareness. Maybe you feel a little more tired after introducing a new herb, or your gut feels mildly unsettled. Perhaps you notice resistance, emotional, physical, or logistical, to a new routine. These yellow lights are invitations to slow down, reassess, and proceed gently. They often pass as the body integrates new inputs. But they shouldn't be ignored.

Red lights, on the other hand, are clear warnings. These include a sudden flare in symptoms, panic, nerve pain, head pressure, overwhelming fatigue, or a sharp return of old neurological sensations. You might find yourself unable to sleep, losing appetite entirely, or feeling emotionally frozen. If your body starts to feel chaotic, unsafe, or "too much," it's time to stop, not push. Something in your current approach is outpacing your body's ability to respond.

In these moments, the priority is rebuilding safety, physically and emotionally. That means increasing hydration, reintroducing grounding foods, resting, and leaning into the tools that help you settle. Once your terrain has reestablished its footing, you can begin again, slowly, and with greater alignment.

This practice of listening doesn't just help you avoid setbacks. It builds trust, in your body, in your intuition, and in the process itself. Over time, you'll begin to sense more clearly what works for you, and what doesn't. You'll move from following a plan to co-creating one.

The terrain is not silent. It's always communicating. When you learn to honor its signals, not fear them, you stop chasing healing and start embodying it.

Healing at the Pace of Safety

Pushing too fast may look like "healing," but often triggers regression or shutdown.

Going too slow may stall momentum, but intentional pacing is not stagnation.

How to adjust:

Flare? Slow down, support drainage, return to nourishment.

Clarity or ease? Add the next layer gently.

Healing led by the nervous system allows deep, sustainable change.

You Are the Steward of Your Terrain

No book, no protocol, and no practitioner can ever know your body the way you do.

This book offers a framework. A compass. A lantern to help you find your way through the fog. But at the end of the day, you are the one walking the path. You are the steward of your terrain.

You are the one who feels the shifts, subtle or strong. The one who knows when sleep deepens or becomes fragmented. When the body starts to soften or harden. When energy rises or drains. These changes don't always show up on labs or checklists. But they are real, and they matter. And you are the one who gets to honor them.

As you move forward, your map will change. It's meant to. You will not stay in the same phase forever. The work you're doing now, stabilizing blood sugar, repairing the gut, calming the nervous system, will open the door to new levels of repair, regeneration, and resilience.

Your terrain will evolve:

As the seasons shift and your needs adjust
As symptoms begin to quiet or transform
As new insight, tools, or support arrive

Sometimes, you may need to circle back to earlier foundations. This is not regression. This is the wisdom of someone who is listening, someone who knows that healing is not linear, but cyclical. You may revisit mineral repletion or drainage even after you've moved into deeper phases. You may return to nervous system work after detoxing. That's not starting over. That's integration.

The goal here is not to reach a finish line. There is no singular "cure," no ultimate destination where all healing is complete and static. The real goal is to build a terrain that doesn't break under pressure, a terrain that flexes, rebounds, adapts. A body that can respond to life with intelligence, not overwhelm.

Every time you choose rest instead of pushing, nourishment instead of depletion, trust instead of fear, you strengthen that terrain. You're not just following a plan. You're rewriting the way your body relates to stress, repair, and resilience.

Trust your timing. Trust your instincts. Own your map.

You are not passive in this process. You are powerfully involved. And every step you take toward safety, rhythm, and inner coherence makes a lasting difference, not just in your symptoms, but in your foundation.

Appendix A: Working with Your Doctor and Tracking Labs

Communicating Your Approach in Clinical Settings

Introducing Terrain-Based Healing to a Practitioner

Frame your approach as complementary, not oppositional.

Emphasize goals: stability, mitochondrial support, inflammation reduction.

Use language familiar to your doctor: "reducing systemic inflammation," "supporting drainage pathways," "targeting nutritional deficiencies."

Keep focus on symptom tracking and functional improvements, energy, bowel regularity, sleep, mood.

Building Collaborative Language

Ask your doctor to help monitor labs related to inflammation, nutrient status, and detox capacity.

Frame interventions as nutritional or lifestyle-based, not "alternative medicine."

Use non-threatening phrases like:

"I've found that tracking certain symptoms helps me understand my energy fluctuations."

"I'd like to make sure we're keeping an eye on my liver and kidney function as I start mitochondrial support."

What to Avoid

Avoid overwhelming your practitioner with complex protocols, simplify your main concerns.

Avoid language that implies distrust or confrontation.

Avoid expecting your doctor to understand or endorse every terrain method.

Suggested Labs to Establish a Terrain Baseline

Establishing a clear baseline helps guide safe repletion, targeted detox, and terrain recalibration. Not all labs need to be run at once, but they can help uncover silent burdens, assess nutrient status, and track healing progress over time. The following list is divided into minimum core labs and optional functional panels, depending on clinical presentation and available resources.

Minimum Core Labs

(Recommended at start of healing process and annually thereafter)

CBC with Differential: Screens for infections, anemia, and systemic inflammation.

CMP (Comprehensive Metabolic Panel): Assesses liver and kidney function, glucose, and electrolytes.

hs-CRP and ESR: Measures silent inflammation and terrain-wide immune activation.

Vitamin D (25-OH D): Essential for immune modulation and mitochondrial biogenesis.

B12, Folate, Homocysteine: Evaluates methylation, nerve health, and detox capacity.

Magnesium (RBC): Intracellular magnesium status (superior to serum levels).

Zinc and Copper: Assesses mineral balance affecting immunity and mitochondrial enzymes.

Optional / Functional Labs

(Add as needed based on symptoms, history, or therapeutic phase)

Ferritin + Full Iron Panel: Monitors iron dysregulation, which can drive oxidative stress and pathogen proliferation.

Thyroid Panel (TSH, Free T3, Free T4, Reverse T3): Critical in fatigue, metabolic slowdown, and chronic inflammation.

Organic Acids Test (OAT): Offers insight into mitochondrial performance, vitamin status, detox capacity, and gut microbial imbalance.

Stool Testing (e.g., GI-MAP, Genova GI Effects): Especially useful for persistent digestive symptoms or suspected dysbiosis.

Mold/Mycotoxin Testing (RealTime, Mosaic/Great Plains): Essential when mold exposure, chronic sinus issues, or environmental illness is suspected.

Heavy Metals (Hair, Urine with Provocation): Only once detox pathways are open and dental amalgams are removed.

Food Sensitivity and Allergy Testing

(Useful for mapping immune burden and guiding early dietary changes)

IgG Food Sensitivity Panel: Measures delayed immune responses and oral intolerance patterns, especially helpful in cases of leaky gut, autoimmunity, MCAS, or neuroinflammatory terrain.

Recommended labs: Mosaic Diagnostics, Vibrant Wellness, US Biotek, ImuPro

Avoid: Generic at-home kits lacking subclass breakdowns or proper antigen prep

IgE Allergy Panel: Screens for acute, anaphylactic reactions to common allergens (e.g., shellfish, peanuts, pollen), especially if a history of severe allergy exists.

Monitoring Detox Safety

GGT (gamma-glutamyl transferase): glutathione depletion marker.

AST, ALT, bilirubin: liver status.

BUN, creatinine, eGFR: kidney function.

Uric acid: inflammation and detox strain.

Ammonia (if available): protein metabolism and detox overload clue.

How to Track Terrain Progress
Symptoms to Monitor Over Time

Energy level (AM/PM)

Bowel movements (frequency, ease, completeness)

Sleep quality (depth, restfulness, vivid dreaming)

Mood/emotional resilience

Skin (rashes, itching, temperature changes)

Cognitive clarity, word-finding, focus

Muscle recovery and movement capacity

Sensitivities (to food, light, sound, supplements)

Breath quality (air hunger, sighing, tension)

Tools for Personal Tracking

Terrain Log: a daily or weekly log of 5–10 core symptoms.

Progress Graphs: chart improvements or regressions across major systems.

Lab Timeline: record date, values, and interpretation of key labs in a spreadsheet or folder.

Flare Journaling: track new symptoms or flare-ups with context (food, stress, weather, supplements).

Signs You're Moving in the Right Direction

Fewer reactive symptoms to environment or food.

More consistent digestion and elimination.

Reduced volatility in mood or physical symptoms.

Increased tolerance to gentle interventions (e.g., lymph work, supplements).

Slow and steady return of functions that had previously declined (e.g., swallowing ease, speech clarity, fine motor control).

Appendix B: Core Therapeutics by Terrain Phase

This appendix groups terrain-based supplements, foods, and herbal supports according to your current healing phase. These are not meant to be taken all at once. Use them like tools, selectively, and in alignment with your terrain's current capacity.

Phase 1: Stabilize & Replete

Goals:

Rebuild baseline energy, nervous system calm, blood sugar balance, bowel regularity, and electrolyte hydration.

Core Nutrients & Foods

Magnesium (glycinate, malate, or threonate): Calms nerves, improves bowel movements, supports mitochondrial function.

Potassium (citrate or from coconut water powder): Restores intracellular hydration, supports adrenal rhythm.

Trace minerals: Sea minerals or shilajit to replenish terrain-wide micronutrient gaps.

Vitamin C (buffered or liposomal): Antioxidant, adrenal-nourishing, supports collagen and immune resilience.

Electrolyte drinks with sea salt: Supports hydration and nerve-muscle signaling.

Egg yolks, bone broth, cooked root vegetables, grass-fed meats: Foundational terrain foods rich in fat-soluble nutrients and glycine.

Supportive Herbs

Ashwagandha: Nervous system calming and thyroid

modulating.

Lemon balm: Calms anxious states, supports gentle viral balance.

Cautions & Notes

Avoid pushing detox or immune-stimulating herbs here.

Begin with food-based supports if supplements are not tolerated.

Focus on sleep, bowel regularity, and circadian rhythm first.

Phase 2: Seal the Gut–Brain Axis

Goals:
Heal gut lining, reduce histamine and immune flares, stabilize neuroimmune signaling.

Core Nutrients & Foods

L-glutamine: Fuel for intestinal cells; strengthens tight junctions.

Zinc carnosine: Repairs gut epithelium, reduces inflammation.

Colostrum (if tolerated): Immune-modulating, promotes mucosal repair.

Quercetin: Calms histamine and mast cell reactivity.

Glycine: Found in broth, also available as a supplement; supports gut lining and neurotransmitter balance.

Cooked squash, ghee, steamed greens, wild blueberries: Soothing, antioxidant-rich foods.

Supportive Herbs

Slippery elm, marshmallow root: Mucosal soothing and gut

lining protective.

Chamomile, peppermint: For gentle digestive calm and bloating relief.

Licorice root (DGL): Gut-soothing and cortisol-modulating (use caution with hypertension).

Cautions & Notes

Introduce new supports slowly, 1 at a time over 3–5 days.

Monitor for food sensitivity flares (e.g., bloating, skin, mood changes).

Nervous system safety (breath, somatic practices) must parallel gut repair for full benefit.

Phase 3: Drain & Detox

Goals:
Open drainage pathways (bowels, liver, kidneys, skin, lymph) before any toxin mobilization.

Core Nutrients & Foods

Glutathione (liposomal or precursors like NAC): Master antioxidant and detox cofactor.

B-complex (with B1, B6, methylfolate, B12): Supports methylation and nervous system detox handling.

Bitters (gentian, artichoke, dandelion): Stimulate bile and liver flow.

Activated charcoal or citrus pectin: Bind toxins in the gut for safe removal.

Beets, lemon water, high-fiber vegetables: Promote bowel motility and bile thinning.

Supportive Herbs

Milk thistle, burdock root: Liver protective and detox-supportive.

Red clover, cleavers: Gentle lymph movers.

Nettle leaf: Nourishes kidneys and reduces inflammation.

Lymphatic and Drainage Therapies

Castor oil packs

Foot soaks with bentonite or Epsom salt

Dry brushing and gentle fascia release

Cautions & Notes

Do not begin chelation until Phase 1 and 2 are solid.

Always bind before or alongside mobilization.

Watch for flare signs (see Detox Chapter); stop if new neurological symptoms appear.

Phase 4: Infection & Immune Reset

Goals:

Gently reduce stealth pathogens only once terrain is stable. Avoid immune overwhelm.

Core Nutrients & Foods

Monolaurin (from coconut): Antiviral, safe for many terrains.

Olive leaf, andrographis, cat's claw: Target bacterial and viral pathogens.

Garlic (aged or fresh): Broad-spectrum support and bile flow enhancer.

Biofilm disruptors (NAC, serrapeptase): Unmask hidden pathogens for immune access.

Herbal infusions (e.g., lemon balm, echinacea): Gentle immune modulation.

Supportive Herbs

Cryptolepis: Powerful antimicrobial (use pulsed).

Lomatium: Potent antiviral (must be respected; possible rash).

Licorice root (for EBV and HHV-6): Immune support and cortisol regulation.

Cautions & Notes

Always pulse antimicrobials: 3–5 days on, 2–3 days off.

Start with antivirals before antibacterial herbs.

Don't begin this phase if bowel, sleep, or emotional stability are impaired.

Phase 5: Regeneration & Repair

Goals:
Promote neuroplasticity, vagal tone, trauma release, and cellular regeneration.

Core Nutrients & Foods

Lion's mane mushroom: Nerve growth factor (NGF) stimulator.

Magnesium threonate: Crosses BBB, supports brain repair.

Phosphatidylserine and phosphatidylcholine: Cell membrane and brain support.

Omega-3s (EPA/DHA): Reduce neuroinflammation and support neuron integrity.

Bacopa, gotu kola: Traditional neurotonics with brain-calming effects.

Fermented foods, medicinal mushrooms, mineral-rich broths: Microbiome and terrain nourishing.

Supportive Practices

Limbic retraining (DNRS, Primal Trust)

Somatic therapy, breath retraining

Nature immersion, sound/vibration therapy

Cautions & Notes

Regeneration requires energy, do not attempt if terrain is still inflamed.

Emotional detox may surface here, ensure support systems are in place.

Avoid combining too many neuroactive agents at once, go slow.

Appendix C: Food Strategy and Therapeutic Meal Frameworks

Food is not just fuel, it's information. The right foods calm inflammation, rebuild the gut, and nourish mitochondria. This appendix offers a phased, flexible framework for building meals that support terrain repair at every stage.

Common Terrain Triggers to Minimize or Eliminate

Inflammatory or Immune-Disrupting Foods

Gluten (especially wheat): Drives zonulin and gut permeability

Casein (dairy protein): Cross-reactive with gluten; can inflame the gut-brain axis

Soy: Often GMO and hormone-disruptive

Corn: High in mold and glyphosate; common cross-reactor

Industrial seed oils (canola, soybean, sunflower): Pro-inflammatory, oxidative

Refined sugar and alcohol: Feed candida, suppress immunity, worsen histamine

Conditional Triggers (based on symptom response)

Eggs: Immune trigger in some gut-inflamed individuals

Yeast/fungi (vinegar, mushrooms): May worsen mold/candida terrain

Nightshades (tomatoes, peppers, potatoes): Can exacerbate joint, nerve, or mast cell issues

High-histamine foods: See below

Meal Templates by Terrain Phase
Phase 1: Stabilize & Replete

Goal: Gentle, easy-to-digest meals with electrolytes, fats, and soft proteins

Template:

Base: Bone broth or veggie broth

Protein: Slow-cooked meats, egg yolk, soft fish

Carbs: Root veggies, squash, organic potatoes or rice (if tolerated)

Fat: Ghee, coconut oil, olive oil

Herbs: Ginger, turmeric, fennel

Sample Meal:

"Nervous system broth bowl": Lamb broth, carrots, zucchini, olive oil drizzle, shredded chicken

Phase 2: Seal the Gut–Brain Axis

Goal: Strengthen mucosal barriers and calm reactivity

Template:

Base: Steamed/roasted low-FODMAP vegetables

Protein: Turkey, wild fish, pastured meats

Binder: Ground flax, chia, seaweed, aloe

Supplement: Glutamine powder in herbal tea

Sample Meal:

"Gut-calm plate": Baked turkey, roasted butternut squash, sautéed bok choy in ghee

Phase 3: Drain & Detox

Goal: Support bile flow, fiber intake, and binder synergy

Template:

> Bitter greens + fiber: Dandelion, arugula, beet greens
>
> Detox boosters: Beets, lemon, apple, radish
>
> Hydration support: Mineral water, cucumber, chia
>
> Optional binder timing: Charcoal or pectin 1 hour away from food

Sample Meal:

> "Liver light plate": Sautéed beet greens, roasted beets, lemon-olive oil sardines

Phase 4: Infection & Immune Reset

Goal: Starve pathogens gently, nourish mitochondria and immune tone

Template:

> Protein-focused: Grass-fed meats, wild fish, organ meats
>
> Antimicrobial sides: Garlic, onion, turmeric, oregano
>
> Low-starch vegetables: Cauliflower, spinach, celery
>
> Optional pulse: Coconut yogurt with monolaurin

Sample Meal:

> "Immune support plate": Bison burger, garlic spinach, steamed zucchini with olive oil

Phase 5: Regeneration & Repair

Goal: Nourish brain and nerve tissue, support BDNF and neurogenesis

Template:

Neuro-fat focus: Salmon, anchovies, eggs (if tolerated), walnuts

Polyphenols: Blueberries, pomegranate, green tea

Herbal tonics: Lion's mane, bacopa, medicinal mushrooms

Warming sides: Steamed roots, turmeric golden milk

Sample Meal:

"Brain regen bowl": Wild salmon, mashed sweet potato, sautéed broccoli in coconut oil

Low-Histamine and Mucosal-Supportive Food Strategies
Low-Histamine Tips

Choose meats frozen at slaughter (avoid aged, cured, smoked)

Avoid fermented foods (sauerkraut, kombucha, vinegars) during flare

Rotate foods to avoid sensitization

Cook and eat fresh (no leftovers >24 hrs)

Use DAO-supportive herbs: Holy basil, stinging nettle, quercetin

Mucosal-Supportive Foods

Slippery foods: Okra, aloe, chia gel

Gelatin-rich broths (slow-simmered bones or skin-on poultry)

Butternut squash, marshmallow root tea, zinc-rich pumpkin seeds

Steamed pears or apples (soothing for gut and lungs)

Substitutions and Ingredient Swaps

As you adjust your meals to support healing, you don't have to give up taste or variety, you just need smart swaps that keep the terrain calm. Below are common food triggers and how to replace them with gentler, nutrient-dense alternatives:

If you're avoiding gluten-containing flours, reach for grain-free options like cassava flour, coconut flour, tigernut flour, or almond flour. These still allow for baking and cooking without triggering zonulin release or gut inflammation.

To replace cow dairy, especially if you're sensitive to casein or lactose, consider using ghee, which is clarified and typically well-tolerated. Some people also do well with A2 protein dairy, particularly from sheep or goats, though this varies by individual.

Corn, which can be highly inflammatory and mold-contaminated, can be swapped with whole, gluten-free grains like millet or sorghum, or better yet, low-starch root vegetables like sweet potato, turnip, or parsnip.

Instead of soy sauce, which contains both soy and gluten, you can use coconut aminos, a fermented coconut product with a similar salty, umami flavor that's free of major allergens.

If nightshades like tomatoes, peppers, and eggplant cause joint pain, nerve irritation, or histamine flares, opt for substitutes like zucchini, celery root, or gently steamed greens to build out your meals.

For recipes that call for vinegar, especially if you're dealing with mold, histamine, or gut issues, lemon juice is a safer acidic alternative. You can also use fresh herbs and olive oil to brighten dishes without triggering symptoms.

In baked goods, eggs can be replaced by plant-based binders like a flax "egg" (1 tbsp ground flax mixed with 2.5 tbsp water), chia gel (same ratio), or a gelatin egg, which also adds gut-supportive amino acids.

To sweeten without driving inflammation, replace refined sugar with small amounts of raw honey (if tolerated), stevia, or monk fruit extract. These are less likely to spike blood sugar or feed pathogens.

And finally, for cooking oils, avoid canola and other industrial seed oils, which are oxidative and highly processed. Instead, use olive oil for cold dishes, avocado oil or ghee for moderate heat, and beef tallow for high-heat cooking.

These substitutions support your terrain while keeping meals satisfying, flavorful, and functional. Over time, these choices retrain your palate and reduce inflammatory load without creating food anxiety.

Appendix E: Terrain Troubleshooting and Symptom Feedback

Healing is not linear, and the path isn't always smooth. This appendix helps you interpret what your body is telling you so you can adjust safely, stay grounded, and know when to pause or pivot.

Sample Roadmaps: Gentle vs. Resilient Start (3-Month Comparison)

Gentle Start (For Sensitive, Advanced, or Collapsed Terrain)

Month 1:

> Focus on hydration, blood sugar, and emotional regulation
>
> Begin mineral repletion (magnesium, sea salt, potassium-rich food)
>
> Add gentle digestive supports (bitters, teas, broth)
>
> Observe bowel patterns and sleep quality

Month 2:

> Begin basic gut repair foods (glutamine, colostrum if tolerated, mucilaginous herbs)
>
> Add low-dose binders away from meals (citrus pectin or chlorella)
>
> Begin light fascia work and foot soaks

Month 3:

> If energy and mood are stable, introduce gentle detox tools (castor oil packs, lemon water)
>
> Trial food-based antimicrobials (garlic, oregano, coconut oil) only if terrain is calm

No chelation, no intense antimicrobials, no pathogen pulsing

Resilient Start (For Early or Robust Terrain)
Month 1:

Same foundations: hydration, sleep, minerals

Begin basic gut repair and drainage together

Add mitochondrial support (CoQ10, B vitamins)

Introduce gentle binders and daily bitters

Month 2:

Begin safe detox layers: sweating, castor packs, red light

Add food-based chelators (cilantro, seaweed)

Start pulsing gentle antivirals if symptoms align (e.g., monolaurin, lemon balm)

Month 3:

Progress to rotating antimicrobials, more potent drainage supports

Continue to assess for flare patterns and nervous system cues

Consider neural repair tools (lion's mane, vagus nerve work)

How to Interpret Symptom Flares

Green Light Symptoms (Signals that indicate healing is progressing):

Brief fatigue followed by increased clarity

Temporary skin breakout that resolves without new triggers

Emotional release followed by calm

Increased urination or stool frequency, then stabilization

Yellow Light Symptoms (Caution, watch and adjust if needed):

Headaches, mild nausea, or gas with new supplement or food

Trouble sleeping after lymph work or detox stimulation

Mood agitation after antimicrobial start

Mild increase in twitching or tingling without panic

Red Light Symptoms (Stop, reassess, and stabilize):

Sudden return or worsening of core neurological symptoms

Burning in the head or spine, panic, dread, or inner heat

Skin rashes that spread quickly, or insomnia that escalates

Constipation, freezing, or crash states after pushing too fast

What to Do When Detox Backfires
Step 1: Stop the aggravating input

Cease any new supplement, antimicrobial, or binder

Pause all detox stimulation (sweating, castor packs, etc.)

Step 2: Rebuild foundation

Increase hydration with minerals

Return to gut-calming foods (broth, squash, gelatin, pears)

Support bowel movement with magnesium, teas, bitters

Ensure nervous system calm: breathwork, grounding, fascia compression

Step 3: Resume slowly

Once sleep, energy, and emotional tone are stable again

Reintroduce one tool at a time, starting with drainage

Herxheimer Reaction vs. Healing Response

Herxheimer (Die-off or Detox Overload):

Sudden onset

Anxiety, tremors, headache, body pain

Heat, pressure, rashes, "poisoned" feeling

Often associated with antimicrobial use or chelation

Can mimic ALS progression, proceed with extreme caution

Healing Response:

Gradual shift, followed by improvement

Short fatigue spike followed by mental clarity

Gentle emotional release, then calm

No worsening of neurological function

Feels like a "wave" rather than a storm

Nervous System Pacing Cues

Listen for safety, not productivity. The nervous system gives clearer signals than symptoms alone when terrain is overwhelmed.

You are in safe healing rhythm when:

You feel grounded or neutral after meals

You sleep deeply and dream

You respond to stress with resilience, not collapse

You feel warmth in hands and feet, digestion feels active

You're able to engage without withdrawing

You are pushing too fast when:

You feel wired but exhausted

Thoughts race or feel invasive

Your body becomes cold, tight, or dissociative

You avoid touch, sound, or light

Emotional outbursts or numbness return

Use your nervous system, not your ambition, as your pacing tool. Safety builds resilience. Resilience rebuilds terrain.

Appendix F: Glossary and Terrain Terms Made Simple

This glossary translates complex clinical language into simple, clear concepts. It is designed to help both patients and caregivers follow the terrain-based model of healing without getting lost in jargon.

A–C

Adrenal dysregulation
A stress-related state where the body's production of cortisol (a hormone) becomes erratic, leading to fatigue, poor sleep, and inflammation.

Antimicrobials
Natural or pharmaceutical agents that weaken or kill microbes like bacteria, viruses, fungi, or parasites. In terrain healing, they are used cautiously and only when the body is ready.

Antioxidants
Compounds that neutralize oxidative stress, damage from unstable molecules called free radicals. They help protect mitochondria and brain cells.

Binders
Substances that bind to toxins in the gut and escort them out through stool. Used to make detoxification safer by reducing toxin reabsorption.

Biofilms
Sticky layers made by pathogens (like Lyme or candida) to hide from the immune system. These films protect microbes from herbs, antibiotics, and immune attack.

Blood-brain barrier (BBB)
A protective shield that separates the brain from circulating toxins

and immune triggers in the blood. When "leaky," it allows inflammation into brain tissue.

Chelation
A chemical process that pulls heavy metals (like lead or mercury) out of the body. It must be done carefully and never before drainage is working well.

Circadian rhythm
The body's 24-hour internal timing system that controls sleep-wake cycles, detox timing, hormone rhythms, and immune activity.

Constellation symptoms
A group of related symptoms that reflect an underlying terrain pattern, such as fatigue, brain fog, and bloating indicating gut-brain axis dysfunction.

D–G

Detox reaction ("Herxheimer" reaction)
A flare or worsening of symptoms when toxins are released faster than the body can eliminate them. Often mistaken for disease progression.

Drainage
The body's natural waste-removal pathways: lymph, liver, bowels, kidneys, skin, and breath. Drainage must be open before detox or antimicrobials are used.

Dry brushing
A gentle brushing technique that stimulates lymph movement through the skin. Helps reduce stagnation and promote detox.

Epigenetics
How the environment, diet, stress, and toxins influence which genes are turned on or off, without changing your DNA code.

Fascia
The web-like connective tissue that wraps every muscle, organ, and nerve. Fascia stores trauma and affects both movement and immune flow.

Foot soaks
Immersing feet in warm water (with salt or clay) to promote circulation, calm the nervous system, and aid gentle detox through the skin.

Glial cells
Immune-like support cells in the brain and spinal cord. They protect neurons but can also release inflammatory chemicals when activated.

Glial priming
A state where glial cells have become hypersensitive, overreacting to even small toxins or stressors, leading to chronic inflammation in the nervous system.

Grounding
Touching the earth or focusing on body sensations to calm the nervous system. Helps shift out of "fight or flight."

H–M

Herx reaction
Short for Herxheimer reaction. A sudden symptom flare during detox, often due to microbial die-off or toxin mobilization. See "Detox reaction."

Histamine intolerance
A terrain issue where the body struggles to break down histamine, causing symptoms like rashes, anxiety, insomnia, or food sensitivity.

Limbic system

A part of the brain involved in emotion, memory, and survival response. Overactivation can lead to chronic fear, fatigue, or illness loops.

Lymphatic system
A drainage and immune system made of fluid channels and nodes that move toxins, pathogens, and waste out of tissues.

Mast cells
Immune cells that release histamine and other chemicals in response to danger. In terrain collapse, they can become overactive, creating inflammation and hypersensitivity.

Methylation
A cellular process required for detox, mood regulation, and DNA repair. Dependent on B vitamins and nutrient availability.

Microglia
Special glial cells in the brain that act like first responders. They protect neurons but can become chronically overactivated.

M–Z

Mitochondria
The "batteries" inside cells. They produce energy and regulate inflammation. Mitochondrial dysfunction is central to ALS terrain collapse.

Mycotoxins
Toxins released by mold. Even after mold is removed, mycotoxins can stay in the body and disrupt mitochondria, brain function, and immune response.

Neuroinflammation
Inflammation inside the brain or spinal cord. Often caused by infections, toxins, or glial overactivation, not just immune imbalance.

Oxidative stress
Damage caused by unstable molecules called free radicals. Can injure mitochondria, DNA, and nerve cells unless balanced by antioxidants.

Parasympathetic state
The "rest, digest, and repair" mode of the nervous system. Healing happens in this state, not in "fight or flight."

Pacing
Slowing or adjusting the healing process to match what the body can tolerate. Prevents crashes and allows sustainable repair.

Priming
A term used when cells (especially immune or glial cells) are in a heightened state of reactivity, more likely to overrespond to minor stimuli.

Redox balance
Short for "reduction-oxidation," the balance between oxidative stress and antioxidant defenses. Critical for brain and mitochondrial health.

Terrain
The body's internal environment, including energy, immunity, drainage, stress response, and toxin load. Healing the terrain means restoring its rhythm, safety, and flow.

Vagal tone
The strength and responsiveness of the vagus nerve, which helps regulate digestion, inflammation, and emotional state. Low vagal tone is linked to poor healing and high stress.

Appendix G: Caregiver and Partner Support

You don't have to carry this alone. And you can't. This appendix is for the partners, family members, and friends walking beside someone with ALS. Your support matters, but it must be sustainable. This is about resilience, not rescue.

Encouragement and Emotional Boundaries
You Are a Mirror, Not a Fixer
Your calm presence can steady the nervous system of your loved one more than any protocol ever could. But the terrain journey is theirs, not yours to solve.

> Offer grounded presence, not pressure
>
> Reassure without overriding autonomy
>
> Let them set the pace, even if it feels slow

Grief and Hope Can Coexist
You may cycle between sorrow, frustration, and deep care. That's natural. What helps is not denying either pole, but learning to hold both.

> It's okay to grieve the loss of ease, routine, or predictability
>
> And it's also okay to believe in repair and resilience
>
> Neither cancels the other

Boundaries Are an Act of Love
Supporting terrain repair doesn't mean dissolving your own needs.

> Make space for rest, solitude, and emotional recovery
>
> Say no to things that drain you beyond your capacity
>
> Speak honestly, loving truth is more stabilizing than silent

resentment

Regulation During Flare Phases
What Co-Regulation Really Means
The nervous system is not a closed loop, yours and theirs are in constant conversation. When symptoms spike, emotional regulation is just as critical as binders or rest.

Calm tone, slow breath, and safe touch can downshift reactivity

Validation ("This is hard. You're not alone.") is more soothing than solutions

Avoid matching panic with panic, stay rooted even when they can't

Tools to Support Regulation Together
Use somatic and environmental cues to help both systems reset.

Gentle eye contact, synchronized breathing, and still presence

Nature walks, warm compresses, or listening to calming music

Agree on a flare plan: what helps, what doesn't, what to avoid saying

Knowing When to Step Back
Sometimes your presence may overwhelm rather than help. That's not failure. That's a cue to pause.

Offer choice: "Would you like space or company?"

Let them know it's safe to ask for quiet or rest

Return when invited, not when anxious

Burnout Prevention and Emotional Rhythm

Caregiving Is a Long Arc, Not a Sprint

Terrain healing can unfold over months or years. Your role needs to be sustainable, not heroic.

Schedule regular breaks from care tasks

Protect your own morning or evening rituals

Let someone else hold the weight when you're nearing depletion

You Are Allowed to Have Needs

Many caregivers silence their hunger, pain, or frustration because "they're not the one suffering." But mutual well-being matters.

Name your emotions without guilt

Ask for support without shame

Your health supports theirs, it's not selfish to guard it

Emotional Rhythm Builds Resilience

Creating emotional rhythm, daily, weekly, seasonally, restores balance.

Celebrate small wins together

Make room for levity, story, or prayer

Anchor your days with rituals: tea, song, breath, light

Final Words

You are not just a helper, you are part of the healing terrain. When you soften into your own breath, you help theirs deepen. When you hold your center, you give them something to lean on. And when you protect your boundaries, you model what safe healing looks like.

You are not responsible for the outcome. But you are invited to walk beside them, with courage, with love, and with your own feet firmly on the ground.

References and Source Materials

This book was written to be simple, clear, and hopeful. To avoid overwhelming readers, citations have been minimized in the text itself. However, every concept here is rooted in published science, clinical experience, and systems biology.

For a comprehensive list of peer-reviewed sources, mechanistic research, and full citations for all major claims, please refer to the companion book:

"Unbroken Nerves: ALS, Mitochondrial Collapse, and Terrain-Based Medicine"

If you're a practitioner or researcher looking to dive deeper, Unbroken Nerves offers full mechanistic breakdowns, source annotations, and therapeutic footnotes.

Additional Books and Resources

These books and tools complement the terrain-based approach described in Strong Roots. They may offer additional insights into healing, neuroplasticity, chronic illness recovery, and whole-person care:

Stealth Infections, Antivirals, and Herbal Protocols

Herbal Antivirals by Stephen Harrod Buhner
Foundational guide to plant-based antiviral strategies, including EBV, CMV, HHV-6, and influenza

Herbal Antibiotics by Stephen Harrod Buhner
Thorough exploration of herbal antibacterials effective against resistant strains and stealth infections

Healing Lyme (2nd ed.) by Stephen Harrod Buhner
Detailed protocols for Borrelia, Bartonella, Babesia, and co-infections

Beyond Antibiotics by Michael A. Schmidt, Lendon Smith, Keith Sehnert
Terrain-supportive model for infection control

Detoxification, Mitochondrial Function, and Environmental Medicine

The Toxin Solution by Dr. Joseph Pizzorno
Practical overview of environmental toxicants and stepwise detox strategies

Mitochondria and the Future of Medicine by Lee Know, ND
Clear breakdown of mitochondrial decline and how to restore energy metabolism

The Metabolic Approach to Cancer by Nasha Winters, ND & Jess Higgins Kelley
Mitochondrial terrain medicine applied to degenerative disease, highly applicable to ALS terrain

Toxic by Neil Nathan, MD
Deep dive into mold, Lyme, EMF sensitivity, and terrain collapse from stealth pathogens

Clean, Green & Lean by Dr. Walter Crinnion
Accessible look at daily detox and endocrine-disrupting chemicals

Neuroinflammation, Brain Repair, and the Gut–Brain Axis

Why Isn't My Brain Working? by Dr. Datis Kharrazian
Neuroinflammation, leaky brain, gut-barrier breakdown, and functional neurology

Gut and Psychology Syndrome by Dr. Natasha Campbell-McBride
How gut integrity shapes the nervous system and immune response

Grain Brain by Dr. David Perlmutter
Neurodegeneration and inflammation tied to modern dietary triggers

Trauma, Nervous System Safety, and Mind–Body Integration

The Body Keeps the Score by Bessel van der Kolk, MD
How trauma shapes physiology, with implications for nervous system regulation

Accessing the Healing Power of the Vagus Nerve by Stanley Rosenberg
Manual techniques and theory for improving vagal tone and neuroplasticity

When the Body Says No by Gabor Maté, MD
The connection between suppressed emotions, trauma, and degenerative disease

Healing Trauma by Peter Levine
Somatic Experiencing® tools for resolving chronic freeze and restoring resilience

Terrain-Based Healing Systems and Foundational Holistic Models

Healing is Possible by Neil Nathan, MD
Gentle, grounded guide for highly sensitive or chronically ill patients

The Root Cause Protocol by Morley Robbins
Mineral balancing, copper dysregulation, and mitochondrial repair

Body Into Balance by Maria Noël Groves, RH (AHG)
Clinical herbalism organized by body system, terrain-focused

The Biology of Belief by Bruce Lipton, PhD

Cellular response to thoughts, emotions, and epigenetic signaling

Terrain Ten by Dr. Nasha Winters
Comprehensive cancer terrain model with system-by-system parallels to ALS healing

Practitioner-Trusted Tools and Sources

Fullscript: A professional-grade supplement platform where patients can access practitioner-quality formulas. Look for brands like Pure Encapsulations, Integrative Therapeutics, and Designs for Health. You can access it through my provider account found at this link https://us.fullscript.com/welcome/rmcpherson

PubMed (pubmed.ncbi.nlm.nih.gov): A free public database of scientific research articles. Readers can search key terms like "mitochondrial dysfunction," "glutathione ALS," or "mast cell neuroinflammation" to explore the studies behind terrain-based insights.

EWG's Tap Water Database (www.ewg.org/tapwater): Search your ZIP code to identify heavy metals, VOCs, fluoride, and other water contaminants. Essential for planning your water filtration strategy.

EWG Skin Deep (www.ewg.org/skindeep): Database of cosmetic and personal care ingredients. Helpful for reducing chemical exposures through deodorant, toothpaste, lotions, and more.

LabTestAnalyzer.com: A user-friendly site for interpreting common bloodwork in functional ranges. Can empower readers to self-track terrain progress with practitioner support.

Toxtown (via NIH Archives): Although no longer actively updated, this archived educational tool from the U.S. National

Library of Medicine explains common environmental toxins by source (air, home, food, etc.).

Functional Lab & Analysis Tools

Rupa Health: Centralized functional lab ordering platform that partners with major labs (Genova, Vibrant, DUTCH, Great Plains). Practitioners can use this to streamline testing.

Cronometer: A detailed food and nutrient tracking app that goes beyond macros and shows micronutrient levels. Useful for tracking repletion progress.

Oura Ring or WHOOP: Wearable tools that track sleep, HRV, circadian rhythm patterns, and recovery capacity—helpful for terrain assessment.

OMEGA Quant: A mail-in finger-prick test for omega-3 status, useful for those rebalancing inflammation and mitochondrial membrane health.

Toxin & Mold Exposure

RealTime Labs or Great Plains Laboratory: Mycotoxin and environmental toxin testing labs for those navigating mold illness or chemical sensitivity.

EnviroBiomics: Dust-based ERMI and HERTSMI mold testing for home environments.

IQAir or AirDoctor: Trusted brands of high-efficiency air purifiers with VOC and mycotoxin filtration capacity.

Clearly Filtered or Berkey: Advanced water filtration systems that reduce fluoride, heavy metals, PFAS, and pesticides.

Supplement Quality & Research

ConsumerLab.com: Independent lab that tests supplement

quality, label accuracy, and contamination risks. Subscription-based.

Examine.com: Deep-dive research summaries on individual nutrients, supplements, and mechanisms, with references to human studies.

NutrEval by Genova: Comprehensive lab panel to assess nutrient status, mitochondrial metabolites, GI markers, and detox indicators.

Medical Literature & Biomedical Databases

Google Scholar: Broader than PubMed, sometimes catches full-text versions and grey literature.

ResearchGate: Platform where many researchers share full PDFs of their publications directly.

Sci-Hub (controversial but used by many researchers): Allows access to full-text studies behind paywalls.

Patient-Facing Education & Community

Surviving Mold (by Dr. Ritchie Shoemaker): Deep dive into CIRS, mold toxicity, and terrain disruption.

HealingALS.org: Grassroots ALS community and documentary series focused on holistic recovery stories.

Planet Paleo or Weston A. Price Foundation: Trusted for traditional food-based healing practices and nutrient-dense ancestral diets.

Genetic Testing Tools

SelfDecode: Genetic interpretation platform for SNPs relevant to detox, inflammation, methylation, etc.

Genetic Genie: Free tool to interpret methylation and detox

pathways from 23andMe or AncestryDNA raw data.

Promethease: Another raw data tool for exploring health-related genetic variants.

Index

Emotional and Psychological Health (trauma, resilience, emotional regulation)

Pages 51–56

Addresses trauma-informed care, grief, emotional reactivation, and inner terrain repair .

Sleep and Circadian Rhythm

Pages 57–59

Covers light exposure, melatonin signaling, mitochondrial repair during sleep .

Environmental Toxins (heavy metals, mold, pesticides)

Pages 60–63

Highlights fluoride, glyphosate, mycotoxins, and synergistic immune damage .

Therapeutic Supplements (key ones like magnesium, CoQ10, Omega-3)

Pages 64–70

Reviews targeted supplementation, key formulas, dosing considerations .

Nervous System Regulation (vagus nerve, parasympathetic activation)

Pages 71–74

Includes vagal tone repair, craniosacral inputs, and nervous system retraining .

Barriers (gut lining, blood-brain barrier)

Pages 75–78

Discusses barrier integrity, inflammation, permeability, and restoration protocols .

Inflammation (microglia, mast cells)

Pages 79–82

Covers neuroinflammation, histamine burden, chronic immune

priming .

Healing Reactions (Herxheimer, healing responses)
Clarifies reactivation events, misinterpreted flares, and productive symptoms .

Disclaimer

This book is for informational and educational purposes only. It is not intended as a substitute for medical advice, diagnosis, or treatment. The author is not a licensed physician, and the information provided here is based on clinical experience, terrain-based models, published research, and patient-centered strategies.

Always consult with a qualified medical professional before making any changes to your medications, diet, supplements, or treatment plans, especially in complex conditions like ALS.

The reader assumes full responsibility for any actions taken based on the contents of this book. The author and publisher disclaim all liability arising directly or indirectly from the use of this information.

www.ingramcontent.com/pod-product-compliance
Lightning Source LLC
Chambersburg PA
CBHW050649270326
41927CB00012B/2950